LIVING WITH APHASIA

PSYCHOSOCIAL ISSUES

LIVING WITH APHASIA

PSYCHOSOCIAL ISSUES

D. LAFOND, Y. JOANETTE, J. PONZIO,
R. DEGIOVANI, AND M. TAYLOR SARNO

With the collaboration of
Gonia Jarema and Karen Sherman

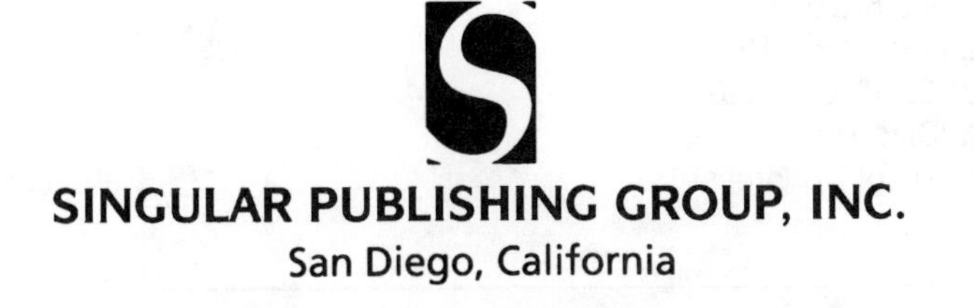

SINGULAR PUBLISHING GROUP, INC.
San Diego, California

Published by Singular Publishing Group, Inc.
4284 41st Street
San Diego, California 92105-1197

Typeset in 10/12 Times Roman by So Cal Graphics
Printed in the United States of America by McNaughton & Gunn

Library of Congress Cataloging-in-Publication Data

Aphasie. English.
Living with aphasia/edited by Denise Lafond . . . [et al.].
p. cm.
Includes bibliographical references and index.
ISBN 1-56593-067-3
1. Aphasia—Psychological aspects. 2. Aphasia—Social aspects.
I. Lafond, Denise. II. Title.
[DNLM: 1. Aphasia—psychology. 2. Self Concept.
WL 340.5–299p]
RC425.A67213 1992
616.85'52'0019—dc20
DNLM/DLC
for Library of Congress

92-49888
CIP

"The aphasia disappears . . .
The person with aphasia remains."

LIST OF CONTRIBUTORS

AUTHORS

Catherine BELIN
Service de neurologie
du Pr. Delaporte
CHU Avicenne
93000 Bobigny, France

Renée BOISCLAIR-PAPILLON
Service d'orthophonie
Hôpital Villa Médica
225, rue Sherbrooke Est
Montréal, Québec H2Y 1C9, Canada

Françoise COT
Centre de recherche
Centre hospitalier Côte-des-Neiges
4565, chemin de la Reine-Marie
Montréal, Québec H3W 1W5, Canada

Christiane CYR-STAFFORD
Service d'orthophonie
Hôpital Marie-Clarac
3530, boul. Gouin Est
Montréal, Québec H1H 1B7, Canada

René DEGIOVANI
59, rue Pascal
83000 Toulon, France

Manfred HERRMANN
Department of Rehabilitation
Psychology
Belfortstr. 16
7800 Freiburg, Germany

Thérèse HIRSBRUNNER
Service d'orthophonie
Hôpital psychiatrique cantonal
2018 Perreux, Suisse

Audrey HOLLAND
Department of Speech and
Hearing Sciences
University of Arizona
Tucson, Arizona 85721, USA

Michelyne D. HUBERT
Centre de recherche
Centre hospitalier Côte-des Neiges
4565, chemin de la Reine-Marie
Montréal, Québec H3W 1W5, Canada

Gonia JAREMA
Département de linguistique
et philologie
Faculté des arts et des sciences
Université de Montréal
& Laboratoire Théophile-Alajouanine
Centre hospitalier Côte-des-Neiges
4565, chemin de la Reine-Marie
Montréal, Québec H3W 1W5, Canada

Yves JOANETTE
Ecole d'orthophonie et audiologie
Faculté de médecine
Université de Montréal
et Laboratoire Théophile-Alajouanine
Centre hospitalier Côte-des-Neiges
4565, chemin de la Reine-Marie
Montréal, Québec H3W 1W5, Canada

Helga JOHANNSEN-HORBACH
School of Speech Therapy
Lorettostr. 2
7800 Freiburg, Germany

Dominique LABOUREL
Service de psychologie
Hospices civils de Lyon
Hôpital neurologique
B.P. Lyon Montchat
69394 Lyon Cedex 3, France

Denise LAFOND
Ecole d'orthophonie et audiologie
Faculté de médecine
Université de Montréal
et Centre de recherche
Centre hospitalier Côte-des-Neiges
4565, chemin de la Reine-Marie
Montréal, Québec H3W 1W5, Canada

Yvan LEBRUN
Neurolinguistiek
Cebouw F R 3
Faculteit Geneeskunde
Laarbeeklaan 103
1090 Brussel, Belgique

André Roch LECOURS
Faculté de médecine
Université de Montréal
et Laboratoire Théophile
Alajouanine
Centre hospitalier
Côte-des-Neiges
4565, chemin de la Reine-Marie
Montréal, Québec H3W 1W5, Canada

Véronique LEFEBVRE-DES-NOETTES-GISQUET
Groupe de Recherche sur les Apprentissages et les Altérations du Langage
(G.R.A.A.L.),
et Centre hospitalier Emile-Roux
94450 Limeil-Brévannes, France

Marie-Andrée LEMAY
Centre de recherche
Centre hospitalier Côte-des Neiges
4565, chemin de la Reine-Marie
Montréal, Québec H3W 1W5, Canada

Pierre Y. LÉTOURNEAU
822, rue Sherbrooke Est
5ième étage
Montréal, Québec H2L 1K4, Canada

Marie-Madeleine MARTIN
Service d'orthophonie
Hospices civils de Lyon
Hôpital neurologique
B.P. Lyon Montchat
69394 Lyon Cedex 3, France

Jean METELLUS
Groupe de Recherche sur les Apprentissages et les Altérations du
Langage (G.R.A.A.L.),
et Centre hospitalier Emile-Roux
48, rue Henri-Barbusse
94450 Limeil-Brévannes, France

Michel PONCET
Service de neurologie et de
neuropsychologie
CHU de la Timone
13385 Marseille Cedex 4, France

Jacques PONZIO
Département de Rééducation du Langage et de Neuropsychologie Clinique
Hôpital Léon Bérard
B.P. 121
83407 Hyères Cedex, France
et 29, rue de la République
Marseille, France

Jacqueline ROLLAND
Service de neurochirurgie
Hôpital Bretonneau
Boul. Tonnelé
37100 Tours, France

Karen SHERMAN
Translator
3875 Plamondon # 9
Montréal, Québec H3S 1K8, Canada

Helen SJARDIN
Royal Perth Hospital
Wellington Street
Perth 6001, Western Australia

Martha TAYLOR SARNO
Department of Rehabilitation
Medicine
NY University School of Medicine
400 E. 34th Street
New York, NY 10016, USA

Philippe VAN EECKHOUT
Service du Professeur F. Chain
Centre du Langage
Groupe hospitalier Pitié-Salpêtrière
47/83, boul. de l'Hôpital
75651 Paris Cedex 13, France
et 11, rue Duvivier
75007 Paris, France

Isabelle VENDEUVRE
Groupe de Recherche sur les Apprentissages et les Altérations du
Langage (G.R.A.A.L.),
et Centre hospitalier Emile-Roux
94450 Limeil-Brévannes, France

Claus-W. WALLESCH
Department of Neurology
Hansastr. 9
7800 Freiburg, Germany

Anne WHITWORTH
Bentley Health Service
Mills Street
Bentley 6102, Western Australia

TABLE OF CONTENTS

SECTION IV — THE PERSON WITH APHASIA AND THE FAMILY

SECTION V — THE PERSON WITH APHASIA AND SOCIETY

To Estelle,
and to anyone who has experienced aphasia,

PREFACE TO THE ENGLISH EDITION

This book was first published in French in 1991 as a first attempt to provide some reflections about different aspects of the personal, familial, and social life of the many persons afflicted with an aphasia. First proposed to Yves Joanette and the other French co-editors by Jacques Ponzio, this venture became more demanding than expected given the range of problems that needed to be covered as well as the influence of cultural factors on the specific ways a given person from a given culture and society experiences aphasia. This is why, in the French edition, contributors were invited from the French-speaking world on both sides of the Atlantic. Researchers and clinicians from Québec, France, Belgium, and Switzerland contributed to the comprehensiveness of the information, reflecting the cultural diversity of the French-speaking world on both personal and legal levels.

In the summer of 1991, with the help of Ana Inès Ansaldo from Argentina, a Spanish edition of this book was made available[1]. Again, the same philosophy was retained. Apart from a translation of most of the chapters from the French edition, several chapters covering differences specific to the Spanish-speaking world were added to the initial core of the book. These chapters provided analogous information relating to aphasia in Spanish-speaking people on both sides of the Atlantic.

The English edition consists of translations of the chapters which appeared in the original French edition, as well as contributions by Drs.

---

[1] Joanette, Y., Lafond, D., Ponzio, J., Degiovani, R., Ansaldo, A. 1991. *El Afasico,* Editorial La Colmena, Laprida 1608, 3A, 1425 Buenos Aires, Argentina.

Manfred Herrmann, Elga Johannsen-Horbach, and Claus-W. Wallesch (in Germany), Drs. Anne Whitworth and Helen Sjardin (in Western Australia), and Dr. Martha Taylor Sarno (in the United States).

One of the dangers of a book such as this one in an unexplored field is to be exposed to some redundancies among chapters. Again, it was felt by the editors that such a redundancy reflecting similar concerns among authors, given that it remains very limited, might stimulate discussion among different authors on a given subject.

It is hoped that this English version, like the French and Spanish editions, will be accessible to a wide audience of people interested in better understanding the person with aphasia. We believe the book is sufficiently sophisticated to satisfy the needs of Speech and Language Pathologists who are knowledgeable about aphasia and its rehabilitation as well as other professionals who work with persons with aphasia. We hope the book will also be valuable to the families and friends of people with aphasia.

It is also hoped that this will be the first of many books devoted to the dissemination of knowledge about the impact of aphasia on the person.

Yves Joanette, Denise Lafond, and Martha Taylor Sarno
Montreal and New York, June 1992

Acknowledgments

The editors are deeply grateful to the authors that contributed to this book. We also want to express our deep appreciation for the work done by Dr. Gonia Jarema and Ms. Karen Sherwin who were in charge of the translation of the French chapters included in this English version. Many thanks to Ms. Thérèse Lafrenière for her careful contribution in typing the manuscript as well as to Ms. Paule Samson for having reviewed the manuscript. Additional thanks to Dr. John H. Ryalls for his invaluable editorial comments.

This book would not have been possible without the continuous support of the Canadian Medical Research Council to Y.J. as well as to the support of the *Fonds de la recherche en santé du Québec* to the *Centre de recherche of the Centre hospitalier Côte-des-Neiges.*

PREFACE

There are aphasias, which have been classified in hundreds of ways from the instructive to the absurd, all reflecting the interests of aphasiologists as much as they do abnormal language behavior. Then there are the persons who acquired aphasia, who cannot be classified except according to their status prior to the illness. To our knowledge, this is the first work which, without being explicitly taxonomical, is devoted entirely to the study of persons with aphasia. The volume thus combines originality and necessity.[2]

There is an abundance of literature on language pathology induced by cerebral lesions. It features many treatises of superb quality which discuss and analyze the various clinical forms of aphasia. In these works the object of study is aphasia rather than the person with aphasia, who often is portrayed as the unwitting carrier of the symptoms rather than as a human being who is transformed by illness. The distinction between having aphasia and being a person with aphasia is essential, and serves as an inspiration for the general perspective of this book.

To focus on persons with aphasia involves an examination of the changes in the persons' private life due to the brain injury, the associated deficits, and their consequences.

It is quite rare that persons with aphasia can put the language problem at a distance in order to analyze and confront it, either alone or with the help of a therapist. Most often, these persons undergo a significant transformation, due not only to the language impairment, but also to the conscious or unconscious intellectual and emotional repercussions of this disorder. Other factors behind the transformation include: motor or sensory disturbances, visual deficits, damage to cognitive functions other than language, and aphasia-related emotional problems.

---

[2] This is a translation of the preface to the original French version of the book.

Obviously, a mere analysis of the symptoms of aphasia will not suffice to pinpoint the problems besetting persons with this condition, especially since two people showing similar anatomical lesions and suffering from identical types of clinical aphasia may manifest strikingly different social behaviors. In other words, a given anatomo-clinical form of aphasia is not categorically associated with a specific personality type. Although there is more than "one" aphasia, this syndrome does transform a person into a distinctive individual.

In this work, persons with aphasia will speak for themselves, so that they can convey their awareness of their deficits. What follow are articles by authors who use their professional experience, testimonies from persons with aphasia and their families, and previously published data to broach an array of topics which will shed light on the self-perceptions of persons with aphasia as well as their relationships with others. The person will be discussed in relation to the illness, the therapeutic context, the family, society, and the law. Several patient profiles illustrate how this disorder dramatically alters these persons' lives.

Neurologists, neuropsychologists, speech language pathologists, occupational therapists, physiotherapists, and anyone who comes into professional contact with persons with aphasia will find that this book sets forth a body of knowledge that had previously been intuitive. Students and researchers in neurolinguistics and psycholinguistics owe it to themselves to read this volume. Those familiar with *L'Aphasie*, published over ten years ago by one of us with François Lhermitte, will surely view this volume as a natural complement. Everyone will appreciate this opportunity to examine in greater detail the person producing the pathological language behavior under study. Furthermore, families of persons with aphasia will now find, in this volume, the answers to many of their questions.

The coordinators of this book, who made invaluable editing contributions, belong to two schools bonded by twenty years of collaboration and friendship. They worked in conjunction with authors from various Francophone countries, all of whom are experienced and recognized in their fields. They deserve our congratulations and gratitude for offering their colleagues an essential and much needed guide for all those who work or live with persons who acquired aphasia.

M. Poncet
A. -R. Lecours

FOREWORD TO THE ENGLISH EDITION

It takes only an hour or so in a good reference library to realize that a staggering amount of study and research has been centered on the problem of aphasia. Perhaps because language appears to be one of the most unique of human characteristics, among the cognitive disorders aphasia has had a disproportionate share of study. It takes longer, but not much, to realize that, although this vast literature has furthered our understanding of the language disorder of aphasia, it has not done very much at all to increase our understanding of the aphasic person. That is, the language disorder is beginning to become a little more transparent, but the persons who have the problem remain relatively unstudied, little understood, still opaque.

In fact, looking at writings on aphasia can result in the notion that individuals with aphasia were deliberately cultivated to increase our understanding of language and its breakdown. There is no comparatively serious effort to understand the effects of the language disorder. This is why this volume is so exciting. Rather than addressing the language deficit, it focuses upon the individuals who have aphasia, their families, and the social issues that result when an individual, previously normal, incurs the loss of language. Although it can be argued that such a perspective results in both a lack of stylistic uniformity and an inevitable smattering of redundancy, these are indeed a small price for readers to pay.

I first encountered this book when it was available only in French. Because I read French miserably, I felt frustrated, even aphasic at the sight of it. This book clearly contained information that transcended the language in which it was written, that could increase our understanding of the aphasic person as he or she exists in western society, at the very least. This English translation is necessarily imperfect in that such a translation adds an inevitable new level of complexity to an already difficult task. Nevertheless it is welcome blessing to the English-speaking aphasic community and their families who seek greater understanding. Just as important, it should be required reading for those who seek to help aphasic persons to overcome their language problems. Finally, it can serve as a resource book for those who study the aphasic condition. Research into the effects of language disorder on people is enriched by this book. Research into aphasic language and what its study can tell us about normal language processing, should be enriched as well.

Audrey L. Holland
University of Arizona
January 2, 1992

INTRODUCTION

Under the guise of civilization, the pretext of progress, we have come to banish from our thoughts anything which rightly or wrongly can be seen as superstition or imaginings; we have prohibited all means of searching for truth that are not in keeping with our customs.
André Breton

This book proceeds from the observation that, apart from a few isolated and exceptional cases, when an individual experiences language impairments following a cerebral lesion, it is the language disorder, the aphasia, that is considered the object of study. The person is seen only as the unwitting host of the syndrome. In this collective work we propose a radically different approach whereby it is the person with aphasia who assumes the lead role. Our aim is to examine, in various ways and from diverse perspectives, the effects of this acquired language disorder on the person.

In other words, we shall study the changes in the lives of people who acquire aphasia as well as its associated problems, such as motor deficits (hemiplegia), sensory and visual deficiencies (hemianopsia), and damage to the cognitive functions other than language (e.g. memory, perception, gestures). These changes can bring about all kinds of difficulties which may be internal in origin or may surface during obligatory interaction with others.

Certain of these problems are discussed in several chapters. We have chosen to leave the texts untouched rather than tamper with them in an effort to avoid repetition. The juxtaposition of the various approaches will provide a multifaceted view of the concepts in question.

In this work, we aim to reveal the diverse psychological, social, and mental repercussions of aphasia. As well, we shall provide clinical and psychological proof that the person with aphasia is a unique individual. We shall also elucidate the relationships that exist between these persons and their familial, social, and therapeutic milieus.

Some of the texts published here may give the impression that persons with aphasia shun social contact, that the families of these persons conspire against them, and that therapists are neither knowledgeable nor objective enough to bring about progress. Since the stories presented below are all factual and the “typical” individuals and families are based on genuine data, we must express our admiration to the families who have undergone great hardship, and who, in most cases, have mustered the inner strength to help the person with aphasia by offering exceptional love and courage. As well, we are truly grateful to the many persons with aphasia who, despite their diminished linguistic capacities, were able to help us gain a better understanding of their lives and of life in general.

The first three chapters of this book (Section 1) focus on the feelings of persons with aphasia. The first chapter[1], an introduction to aphasia, contains gripping introspective testimonies by persons who acquired this disorder; men and women who, for various reasons, lost, temporarily or permanently, the capacity to communicate with others by means of language. These comments were compiled by doctors and researchers working with persons with aphasia. Aphasia is thus described in the actual words of the people who were stricken by the illness. The second chapter, complementary to the first, covers the varying degrees of awareness that persons with aphasia have of their illness. There are, in fact, cases where the aphasia manifests itself through varying degrees of unawareness of the problem. This condition clouds the clinical picture and aggravates the effects of the aphasia. The final chapter in this section provides an overview of the physical experience of persons with aphasia, with a discussion of the general effects of aphasia on the individual. Overall, the first three chapters will enable the reader to step into the person’s shoes in order to comprehend better the following chapters which discuss the effects of aphasia on the person.

The second section deals with the effects the syndrome has on the personality of individuals with aphasia. Chapter 4 discusses the psychological effects of aphasia, which are exceptionally traumatic in that these persons’ inability to communicate prevents them from sharing their experience with loved ones. One possible solution lies in nonver-

[1] Given that the English version is not a mere translation of the French edition, the reader will not benefit from a full description of each chapter included in this edition.

bal creative activities, the subject of Chapter 5. In fact, many persons with aphasia have benefitted from engaging in artistic expression, where emotions can be expressed without language. Incidentally, these persons have often been the subject of creative works. Description of persons with aphasia in literature are not only a valuable source of information on the illness, but also shed light on the way they are perceived by those around them.

In the third section the authors examine a particular stage in the life of the person with aphasia — that of rehabilitation. Therapists with extensive experience present their viewpoints on the interpersonal dynamics that aim to foster recovery at the onset of treatment. They also describe attitudes which can foster the person's ability to communicate (Chapter 6). This section also features a discussion of the obstacles to patient management, which are linked to the particular psychological traits of a given group (Chapter 7).

The familial relationships of the person with aphasia are the subject of the fourth section. Two complementary chapters, each from a different context, examine this thorny issue. Chapter 9 describes the European setting, while Chapter 10 offers a North American view of the problem. Despite the differences between the cultures, the two chapters collectively paint a relatively universal picture of the reciprocal relationships between persons with aphasia and their families. They are therefore particularly valuable for anyone who has a family member with acquired aphasia.

The fifth and final section grapples with the question of society and the person with aphasia. In fact, contrary to most illnesses, aphasia gives rise to particular social difficulties for the person who has acquired this syndrome. Chapter 12 discusses the person with aphasia in society. Readers will discover that, despite their significant numbers, these persons have, to date, no recognized social status, unlike victims of many other illnesses. This unfortunate situation is a further setback in their struggle to integrate into society. One particular problem is that of the person with aphasia and the workforce. The person who wants to return to work, or even worse, who is contemplating a new career, is often exposed to a lack of understanding on the part of employers and colleagues. This problem is looked at in Chapter 13, which presents an exclusive study of persons with aphasia who have faced ignorance and intolerance in the workplace. Overall, it is probably in their relation with the law that persons with aphasia experience most acutely the marginalization imposed by society. In fact, as the legal system is based on a series of essentially verbal rules, a person who is deprived of language is particularly disadvantaged. Chapter 14 deals with this aspect of the problem along with specific details regarding codes and rules currently in effect on either side of the Atlantic. This volume concludes with a section that outlines the key role of associations for persons with aphasia in terms of maintaining enduring and rewarding social links. The authors of Chapter 16 summarize the operating methods of these associations and provide the reader with insight into their formation.

Y. Joanette, J. Ponzio, D. Lafond, and R. Degiovani

CHAPTER 1

THE PERSON AND APHASIA

Y. JOANETTE, D. LAFOND, AND A.R. LECOURS

We can't talk. We can't even say it's because we're crazy, but it's because we are sick. If it happened to you, I would go see you. Me, I would know what's happening to you. But others would't be able to understand you.
(L.D.)

Aphasia is not a "rare" syndrome; a stroke, a brain tumor, or a head injury may induce several clinical manifestations, some of which may be directly linked to a person's communicative capacities, i.e. language. When accompanied by a brain injury, disturbances in oral and/or written expression, such as difficulty in understanding the speech of others, recalling the name for things, producing speech, and programming the motor mechanisms required for the proper articulation of words, are collectively known as aphasia.

Aphasia also cannot be considered a "new" disorder. The first clinical definitions appeared late in the 19th century, along with basic descriptions of its typology. In fact, the names of pioneers such as Paul Broca (1865) in France, or Carl Wernicke (1874) in Germany, have come to be associated with specific clinical forms of aphasia.

Although aphasia is neither "rare" nor "new," the contemporary medical and paramedical spheres are generally poorly acquainted with it. Apart from those who work directly with persons with aphasia, for the most part speech pathologists and neurologists, most people are mystified and feel ill-equipped to cope with this disability. These people include physiotherapists, occupational therapists, social workers, nursing staff, family doctors or specialists consulted, and even the friends and family of the person with aphasia. It is crucial that all of these people receive as much information as possible regarding the nature of aphasia, and especially what it means to **have aphasia.** If the truth be told, persons with aphasia are largely misunderstood by those around them. Not too long ago, people with Wernicke's aphasia were considered psychiatric patients and were often committed to insane asylums!

The aim of this first chapter is not to examine aphasia as a pathology, but rather to consider persons with aphasia as human beings who are grappling with a problem that not only reduces or eliminates their capacity to communicate with others, but one which is also often coupled with other physical disabilities such as motor or visual deficits. Furthermore, persons with aphasia often experience family and social problems.

Unlike studies of **aphasia,** where traditionally the "experimental" method is used, studies of **persons with aphasia** can be better approached by using data arising from personal experience. One of the means of gathering this type of data is through introspection, which, in this case, consists of examining one's own illness. For persons with aphasia, the prospect of introspection is often limited. In many cases it is inconceivable to expect people who have reduced command of language (i.e. the ability communicate their impressions) to engage in introspection. Nevertheless, since most persons with aphasia eventually recover full or partial use of their language abilities, introspection is often ultimately feasible. In this exercise, however, some patients are more apt than others.

A further limitation to introspection is its subjective nature. It only reflects the perceptions of one individual suffering from a particular type of aphasia in a particular context. To offset this subjectivity, the introspective comments of a number of people must be studied with a view to detecting common elements. Thus, although this approach lacks the rigor of an objective method, it is interesting and thought-provoking nonetheless.

The primary aim of this chapter is to allow for a better understanding of the thoughts and emotional responses of persons with aphasia. We specifically wish to explore these persons' attitudes towards their communication problems, along with reactions of family members and friends. To this effect, two principal sources of introspective comments will be consulted.

- The first consists of bibliographical sources. Some persons with aphasia who recovered particularly well wrote memoirs. For example, certain doctors who acquired aphasia committed their personal experiences to paper. The earliest known work is that of professor Lordat, Dean of the Faculty of Medicine at Montpellier, who acquired aphasia in 1825. His volume was followed by two publications by Swiss doctors, Dr. Saloz, from Geneva, whose memoirs were published by Professor Naville in 1918, and Dr. Auguste Forel, director of a mental institution in Zurich, who wrote his personal observations in 1927 before becoming a noted entomologist(!). Since then, several other persons with aphasia have produced memoirs, including speech pathologists, psychiatrists, and people from other backgrounds who wanted to recount their experience.

- The clinical milieu is the other source of introspective remarks. The comments were made by patients treated by one of the contributors (D.L.) at the *Centre de rééducation du langage et de recherche neuropsychologique de l'Hôtel-Dieu de Montréal*, and the *Centre de recherche du Centre hospitalier Côte-des-Neiges.* The comments were offered spontaneously, or as responses to suggestions or questions.

After the comments were gathered and tabulated, two categories seemed to suggest themselves:

• Those dealing with communication problems: These comments reflect the persons' intimate thoughts about their language problems. The comments will be presented in terms of the traditional four language modalities: oral and written expression and comprehension.

• Those on the reactions of persons with aphasia to the communication problem. These comments deal with the persons' emotional response to the disability, as well as the reactions of family and friends.

INTROSPECTIVE COMMENTS

As mentioned above, the following comments arise from spontaneous or induced introspection by several persons with aphasia, each of whom is suffering from a particular form of aphasia.[1] Given the significant differences in the symptoms of the various clinical types of aphasia, readers should be forewarned, and should not generalize and attribute a particular comment to all persons with aphasia.

Comments on Language Problems

The introspective comments—the person's perception of his own communication problems—will be categorized in terms of the four modalities of language, the standard reference points in clinical evaluations of aphasia.

Oral Expression

In most cases, aphasia impairs the patient's ability to communicate verbally. One of the most common signs of aphasia is word-finding difficulties. Other symptoms, however, such as difficulty in combining articulatory movements in order to produce the sounds of a language, difficulty in juxtaposing sounds to form words and words to form sentences, are associated with particular types of aphasia.

Especially at the onset of the disorder, persons with aphasia may not necessarily be fully aware of their disability.

"I told [my husband] where to put my rings, and he put them some other place. He really is distracted." (H.W.)

Sometimes person with aphasia become aware of their condition when they observe their difficulty in communicating.

---

[1] Given the aims of this chapter, and in order to facilitate reading, the clinical type of aphasia will not be systematically mentioned for each of the persons with aphasia who have provided comments. For those who are interested, however, all the aphasiological diagnoses of the patients can be found in Table 1–1.

TABLE 1–1
Sources of introspective comments

Initials	Type of Aphasia	Source
A.F.	Wernicke's	"Forrell, A." quoted in, Alajouanine, T. & Lhermitte, F. "Essai d'introspection de l'aphasie", *Revue Neurologique (Paris)*, *110*, No. 6, 609-621, 1964.
A.H.	Unknown	Hall, A. "Return from silence. A personal experience" in *JSHD*, *26*, 174-177, 1961.
C.C.	Paroxystic	Hôtel-Dieu de Montréal (HDM)
C.D.	Unkown	"Dalberg, C.C." in, Dalberg, C.C. & Jaffe, J. (Eds), *Stroke: A Doctor's Personal Story of His Recovery*, New York: W.W. Norton & Co., 1977.
D.C.	Wernicke's	HDM
G.L.	Pure anarthria	HDM
H.W.	Broca's	Wulf, H., *Aphasia, My World Alone*, Detroit: Wayne University Press & Englewood Cliffs, N.J.: Prentice Hall, 1973.
J.B.	Mixed aphasia	HDM
J.L.	Wernicke's	"Lordat, J." quoted in, Alajouanine, T. & Lhermitte F. "Essai d'introspection de l'aphasie", *Revue neurologique (Paris)*, *110*, No. 6, 609-621, 1964.
L.D.	Wernicke's	HDM
M.B.	Unknown	Buck, M. *Dysphasia: Professional Guidance for Family and Patients*, Englewood Cliffs, N.J.: Prentice Hall, 1968.
M.C.	Unknown	Case "C" in, Alajouanine, T. & Lhermitte, F., 1964.
M.R.	Unknown	Case "R" in, Alajouanine, T. & Lhermitte, F., 1964.
S.B.	Unknown	Sies, L. & Butler, R. "A Personal Account of Aphasia", *JSHD*, *28*, 261-266, 1963.
S.S.	Wernicke's (reduced)	"Dr. Saloz" in, Naville, F. "Mémoire d'un médecin aphasique", *Arch Psychol*, *17*, No. 65, 1918.
Y.M.	Broca's	HDM
M.L.	Unknown	"M.L." in, Rolnick, M. & Hops, H.R. "An Aphasia as Seen by the Aphasic," *JSHD*, *34*, 48-53, 1969.
J.J.H.	Conduction	Centre hospitalier Côte-des-Neiges (CHCN)
M.S.	Conduction	CHCN
L.M.	Broca's	CHCN
M.M.D.	Wernicke's	Delezenne, M.M. *Une aphasie vécue*, Unpublished manuscript, 1989.
J.A.	Mixed	CHCN
R.A.	Wernicke's (particularly affecting written language)	Aubin, R. *Le cerveau a ses raisons*, Québec: Editions du Papyrus, 1988.

"I wonder how many questions I've asked [my husband]... Later I learned that I had not tried to talk all afternoon. [He] had tried to answer the questioning in my eyes." (H.W.)

"The first three words that I could utter were: *shit, difficult, eat.* I couldn't think of other words, and it was only when I would see other people's expressions and baffled looks that I realized that there was something wrong." (M.M.D.)

"I didn't realize that I couldn't speak... Dr. B. came. He showed me objects and asked me to name them. I could only nod *yes* or shake my head *no.*" (L.M.)

Other persons with aphasia may experience a more sudden awareness.

"I found that when I wanted to talk, I couldn't recall the appropriate expressions. My thoughts were ready, but I could no longer command the sounds that expressed them. I said to myself *so it's true that I can't speak any more.*" (J.L.)

"I wanted to speak, but no sounds came out of my mouth." (J.A.)

"The telephone rang, I would answer and, much to my surprise, the words would not come out. My voice sounded like an old, broken-down record. At times, I would cry out meaningless utterances." (M.S.)

One person with aphasia noticed that, after some time, he recovered his everyday vocabulary sufficiently, yet abstract language was still inaccessible:

"Bit by bit, I remember simple everyday words, but I am still unable to express an opinion." (L.M.)

For some persons with aphasia, linguistic expression is so disturbed that their oral output becomes meaningless. In these cases, do the persons with aphasia really wish to communicate, or does this babble represent a malfunctioning machine? Below is testimony from a patient who suffers from this problem:

"I *do* want to say something, but I can't find it... Of course, I, I want to talk!" (C.C.)

"When people came to visit, I tried to tell them something, but I was unable to speak one clear word. I chattered, certain that I was understood. It took me a long time to realize that I was unable to understand much, and that others couldn't understand a thing." (M.M.D.)

The words are stuck inside. They can no longer come out easily.

"Naturally, I couldn't talk. I felt *walled in...* I wanted a doctor to listen to me... even if me, I didn't know how to speak."(L.M.)

The person with aphasia does indeed want to say something, but lacks the instrument of communication—language.

"My ideas were fine; it was my psychological tools that were faulty. I lost my symbols, my ability to express thoughts through speech and writing." (S.S.)

"My head bent, my arms crossed, I was racking my brain for what I *knew* was a word." (L.M.)

"My mind gallops happily, but translating thinking into words is a totally different proposition." (H.W.)

"I thought I possessed the normal or ideal mental image of complete words, but I was still plagued by the problem of articulation. For example, I couldn't say the word *'maraschino.'* I would always say *'marachisino'* or *'mascharino'*. I knew that the word began with an 'm' but I couldn't pronounce the other letters in succession." (S.S.)

"My problem was communicating orally, explaining... I had problems forming words." (J.J.H.)

It is well known that despite a considerable impairment of language, the person with aphasia is still capable of near normal linguistic performance when it comes to "language automatisms" such as reciting the days of the week, the months, or certain prayers. Persons who acquire aphasia are well aware of this phenomenon.

"Being religious, I am used to saying the rosary. When I had aphasia, I would often be able to say it." (C.C.)

"When I served mass, I was able to give the answers of the servant, but I didn't know what I was saying, how I said it, and especially, I didn't understand it any more. I was talking, but I didn't know what I was saying... It wasn't me speaking." (M.R.)

"The speech therapist asked me: *Can you count? How high?* I had no problem counting to thirty, but I couldn't go further. *What time is it?* she continued. It was around 11:15, but I didn't know how to say it." (M.M.D.)

Although persons with aphasia are not always aware of the exact nature of the mistakes that slip into their speech, they often do sense the presence of these errors.

"I am well aware that some words don't come out right, but I don't know how I am pronouncing them... I am scared to talk, scared to make silly mistakes." (C.C.)

Persons with aphasia may spontaneously discover coping strategies to handle these difficulties.

"I need to visualize the written word in order to pronounce it properly." (G.L.)

"When I have trouble finding a word, I need to concentrate for a few minutes; I try to think of similar words, and the word will come to me all of a sudden." (M.S.)

"If someone helps me with a syllable, more often than not I can find the word. But if people try to guess the word, I lose track of the whole sentence." (M.S.)

"When I sing, the tune or melody will suggest the words, and I feel my nerve pathways become clearer and messages flow easier." (S.S.)

Incidentally, techniques involving melody are currently used in certain forms of treatment.

There is a basic principle that exudes from these introspective remarks on the difficulties with oral expression: Aphasia does not seem to affect the very essence of the individual, i.e. their thoughts. Rather, aphasia affects mainly the communication mechanism that expresses these thoughts. The comments below bear witness to this viewpoint.

"Forgetting words seems like a shelling of ideas, since the idea loses its concrete envelope, the word. In effect, the two elements lose their mutual and reciprocal bond. What is well thought out is expressed easily (sic)." (S.S.)

"I always was able to imagine objects, but was unable to recall their names. Now, words are more often accessible, on the tip of my tongue. . . but they still don't come quickly. Mind you, I find a way to express the idea in another way." (L.M.)

Oral Comprehension

To comprehend oral language an individual must be capable of extracting a linguistic message from the perceived sounds of the language. In certain types of aphasia, this ability to understand can be disrupted. These patients are usually suffering from a lesion in the posterior (temporal and/or parietal) region of the language center. Persons with this type of aphasia are thus unable to understand what they hear, although their hearing is not impaired (deafness is absolutely not a factor).

"I heard something, and I didn't understand . . . It was like Chinese, or . . . I don't know . . . not a foreign language, but more like something meaningless, how shall I put it, I heard vague words." (C.C.)

"When I speak to someone . . . my brain seems to be spontaneously active, I express myself well enough. But when the other person answers, I am unable to understand what he says. I can't engage in conversation —it's a form of deafness." (M.M.D.)

The person with aphasia who comprehends with difficulty is unable to associate the acoustic representations of words with their referents.

"In my case, I couldn't remember the psychological or mental representation of a word and its acoustic symbol. At times I easily forgot its sound as a verbal symbol, I only could think of an ordinary noise." (S.S.)

Some persons with aphasia who experience oral comprehension loss are able to recognize familiar words but cannot understand them.

"At first, I heard words and I could only recall that I knew them, the act of hearing them did not reveal their meaning to me." (M.C.)

For some patients, if one word is understood, other words can automatically be understood.

"In the same way that I would associate one person with another, a word I would hear would be the key to a whole string of words." (M.C.)

Note that persons with aphasia generally try to understand everything that is said to them.

"I do try to understand, but I can't. I ask myself sometimes, *What does he mean by that?* and I can't understand."(C.C.)

Persons with aphasia are, after all, sentient beings, and even if they can't understand oral expression, they are quite capable of interpreting gestures and tone of voice.

"I don't remember much about the onset of my illness, but even a long time after, I have a bitter memory of the doctor and interns' visits, and the discussions they would have. I didn't understand everything, but I could see by their expressions and their tone of voice that they were not too optimistic about my prognosis." (M.B.)

"On the other hand, I understood gestures and facial expressions. I said to myself: *If they look unhappy, it's because they know a lot about my condition."* (C.D.)

Comprehension disturbances may be less severe depending on the degree of loss and the patient's stage of rehabilitation.

"I could understand simple things, but complicated instructions—not at all." (C.D.)

"I was always able to understand what people were saying, but if several people spoke at once, in loud voices, well, I blocked my ears, and my head hurt . . . I felt the same when it was noisy." (M.S.)

Finally, this response given by a person in therapy, whose comprehension problems had abated considerably:

"When you speak slowly, it's alright; but if you speak too quickly, it's as if I only hear sounds, I can't understand well. It's the same way if I am with a few people, I can't always follow the conversation. By the time I try to understand what was said, two or three other people have already spoken, and I get all confused." (L.D.)

"I must add that my comprehension is nonexistent when a conversation begins, there is an interruption, and the conversation continues." (M.S.)

Written Expression

We were only able to collect a few introspective comments on written expression problems. This may be explained by the fact that persons with aphasia are less worried by a disability that affects written expression, which is a less primal modality than oral expression. It is also possible that many comments on oral expression also apply to written expression.

As in the case of oral expression, some persons with aphasia only become aware of their problems when confronted with an example of their own diminished capacity.

"I felt my left hand move . . . I tried to write: *Where am I?* But all that I could scribble were a few illegible marks."(J.A.)

"When I realized that I was aphonic, my first act was to grab a pencil and paper and to jot down a message; I was unable to do so." (M.S.)

"It just doesn't come, you know? It doesn't come from inside, the way you have to form letters . . . Sometimes, I say to myself, *Hey, but I can write*, and I try, but then I can't." (C.C.)

Even when the writing problem is more subtle, persons with aphasia sense that their performance has deteriorated in relation to their abilities prior to the illness.

"When I'm writing, I may omit letters, syllables, or words at any time. If someone interrupts me while I'm taking a dictation, I am no longer able to continue immediately where I left off. I often forget the beginnings of long sentences, and have to reread them in order to continue in the same vein." (A.F.)

"Only my name was legible at all times and written flawlessly." (M.S.)

"After a few (speech therapy) sessions, I could spell short words; by spelling out loud, it was easier to write." (M.S.)

"Writing long sentences was difficult; the syllables were not in order, or, once I began, I couldn't remember the rest of the sentence. I had to concentrate fully on the words, the grammar, and it was necessary to reread several times." (M.S.)

Here, a person with aphasia attempts to describe her difficulties in written expression and the strategies she used to overcome them.

"How do I try to write? . . . I think, but I must speak out loud all that I write. I am unable to think abstractly the way I used to. I have to hear aloud what I want to express . . . I think while whispering to myself, and I write at the same time. When I read the work over, I make corrections . . . " (M.M.D.)

Certain cases seem rather odd, yet they can be explained by specific deficits affecting grammatical categories.

"It's not the longest and most complicated words that give me the most trouble . . . instead, it's the small words like: 'in,' 'the,' 'her,' 'by,' especially small invariable words and negatives." (S.S.)

Other problems with written expression manifest themselves in isolated examples.

"I can think of the word phonetically, but not written. I just can't. I can say it, I hear it, but I can't see it. Moreover, I don't know the meaning of the word anymore." (A.F.)

Written Comprehension

Some persons with aphasia who have oral comprehension deficits find it difficult to understand written language.

"At the same time as I lost the memory of the sounds of words, I also forgot their written symbols. Syntax was gone. I still could recall the alphabet, but not the way in which letters were used to form words." (J.L.)

"Reading was impossible for at least a couple of months. I couldn't make sense of what I was reading, all the letters seemed to be jumbled together." (M.S.)

"When I read, I often missed important passages, or I would misunderstand the meaning of a sentence." (A.F.)

"When I tried to read a newspaper or magazine, all I could see were meaningless symbols." (M.M.D.)

Awareness of this deficit forces some patients to resort to various compensatory strategies.

"At the onset of my illness, I had to read out loud . . . In order to read, I have to visualize the letter or the word; not only how it looks, but how it sounds . . . People would hear me whispering the letter or the word before uttering it out loud. The problem was that I needed not only to see the form of the letter, but also hear how it sounds." (S.S.)

For some patients, even the size of the letter affects their ability to comprehend what is written.

"If the letters are written in large print, I can read and understand well.

But small print is just too confusing . . . " (D.C.)

Even patients who have recovered well do not find reading as easy as it was before the illness.

"I read, I understand what I read more or less, but I can't remember the plot. Often, I have to look over the chapter again, or reread the previous paragraph to see where I am." (J.B.)

"I can't read because I can't concentrate. Sometimes I even have trouble recognizing letters." (M.S.)

Here, a person with aphasia describes and sheds light on the problems she experiences when reading a newspaper article:

"I open a magazine or a newspaper and I read only the headlines (it is too hard to read an article) and I'm not sure of what I read. For example: 'In Moscow, Gorbachev declares strikes illegal.' Who will declare? *Illegal.* Are these words both negative or both positive? Who will declare?" (M.M.D.)

This final anecdote relates the experience of a person with aphasia who dined at a restaurant:

". . . well, it was a Friday, and I don't eat fish. I never eat fish—I just don't like it. So I went to a restaurant. The waitress hands me the menu, I tried to read it . . . I couldn't read the menu; imagine how I looked! So I point to a line at random . . . The waitress comes back and serves me a plate of fish! And to think, that's the last thing I wanted. Fortunately for me, there were vegetables on the plate. So I ate the vegetables . . ." (C.C.)

Comments on Reactions to the Language Disturbances

The introspective comments below reflect the psychological or emotional reactions of persons with aphasia to their language disturbances. Three aspects of these reactions will be discussed: First, the reaction of the persons to their condition; secondly, reactions within the person's family; and finally, reactions within the health-care environment.

The Self-Perceptions of Persons with Aphasia

Language can be considered the most widely used communication tool. If so, the loss of this tool can induce feelings of isolation and solitude in persons with aphasia. People who are isolated from their peers often experience sadness, frustration, and desperation. Persons with aphasia, unable to express ideas, to communicate through language, are the only ones capable of reading their thoughts.

"You feel like you are in a cave, you hear your voice echoing. You're afraid of human contact, but you don't want to go out alone." (L.M.)

"For over three months, I was in a bleak gray-black desert, barren, no sound, no color . . . insipid, endless, everything was dead." (M.R.)

"That awful feeling of being a prisoner within myself!" (H.W.)

"I felt figuratively imprisoned in a tomb." (S.S.)

"It's absolutely brutal: You still have the same ideas, the same mind. It takes time to get used to, like the loss of an arm." (J.J.H.)

"I'm not the same. But I thought I was the same. My life is a contradiction."

"I can't read, I can't write, I can't speak, and I can't understand . . . at times like these, I really feel miserable." (C.C.)

"I noticed a change in me, I was another person, someone who was unable to express the little I knew, I was ashamed." (M.S.)

"The predominant psychological phenomenon at the onset of my illness . . . was an urgent need and desire to search for psychological explanations for what I considered to be missing . . . why I wasn't despairing. I was always under the impression that I must cling to my will." (S.S.)

Some persons with aphasia experience considerable anguish as a result of their disability and pessimism about the future.

"My life is a mixture of fear and uncertainty. This recent event can only lead to questions, and this terrifies me." (R.A.)

Persons with aphasia tend to avoid communication; they try to disguise their problem.

"Sometimes, the janitor would be away . . . I would be alone at home . . . Once I had to answer the intercom. I said *Hello?* I heard the person speaking on the other end, but I couldn't understand him. So, to prove that it wasn't me who had the problem, I repeated *Hello! Hello! Hello!* as if to signal that the line was bad. That's how I got out of that situation." (C.C.)

"I really just pretend to understand what people are saying! Sometimes I will ask them to repeat, but then I hear another version." (M.M.D.)

An orientation counsellor adds this comment on how aphasia affected his work:

"Through my work, I understood what persons with aphasia are going through, what it's like not to be able to speak. The idea of this immense problem is like having the rug jerked out from under your feet. The voice is silent, but the heart still speaks." (R.A.)

The Person's Feelings towards Family Members

The relationship between the person with aphasia and his or her family and friends is that of an individual isolated from his environment and, all too often, misunderstood.

"I was listening to them from my bedroom. They said *My God, she's going to die,* and they were practically arguing over who would get what of my estate. Me, I could hear them, but I was unable to let them know that I understood what they were saying." (Y.M.)

"When people visited me, I was made aware of my condition because I couldn't greet them with *Hi! How are you today?*" (J.L.)

"Many people came to visit, but I found it annoying trying to talk to people . . . and the visitors were often uneasy." (L.M.)

"I was stepping from one strange world (the hospital) into another (home). To paraphrase two better poets, I was (to my thinking) an island; a stranger, afraid, in a world I never made." (S.B.)

To those who attempted to reassure and help the patient by comparing their disturbances to a foreign language situation, this person with aphasia replied:

"Someone asked me why I don't pretend that I'm trying to speak a foreign language . . . use gestures for example. I think that my problem is different. In French, I know what I have to say . . . but in another language if I don't know the word I can act it out." (L.M.)

Because they did or do have difficulties in communicating through language, persons with aphasia (and sometimes persons who used to have aphasia) often fear being considered inadequate by family members. The aphasia may disappear, but the person with aphasia remains.

"What aggravates me is the trial and error, the self-correction as I'm speaking. I find it tiring to talk for a long time. It seems to me that I don't speak well." (J.B.)

"Everyone was sure that I was progressing because I was speaking better and I was writing letters. They are still saying that, while I personally think that my skills in reading, understanding and arithmetic are not improving at all." (M.M.D.)

"He feels unable to understand the notion of the structure of the word on his own, and is forever tormented by the feeling of having lost some of the elements. As a result, he feels that an outsider cannot understand him." (S.S.)

Consequently, persons with aphasia withdraw into themselves. These persons will subsequently avoid situations where they are expected to communicate.

"If you don't know words, you keep quiet . . . When it's noisy, you can't talk . . . People talk for us . . . Anyway, when we talk, it's not the way it used to be . . . you keep quiet." (L.M.)

"I'm not sure of myself, I feel uncomfortable around other people, I have problems communicating." (J.B.)

"Even while disliking myself, I preferred my own miserable company." (S.B.)

"My interests are mostly solitary—reading, writing, ruminating; I make my own little world . . . living in the midst of people, and yet apart from them, not having much occasion or feeling much need or desire to communicate directly . . . " (S.B.)

Other persons with aphasia crave being surrounded by others:

"I'm only happy when a person close to me is nearby. I need to feel understood, even if I don't say anything." (R.A.)

At times, family and friends may act in ways that are not appreciated by persons with aphasia.

"I want to say something . . . just before I start saying it she helps. Sometimes if she would stay back and let me finish, I would be all right . . . They are trying to express my ideas . . . It's easier for them to think of the word I'm trying to. If I want to work on this particular work . . . they get impatient." (M.L.)

"I feel as if people don't give me enough time to express my ideas fully . . . it's too bad. They jump from one topic to another, just like that . . . two people talk at once, it's awful." (L.M.)

"I feel useless . . . slightly distanced from the family because I can only understand things after some time. My world has shrunk." (M.M.D.)

One person with aphasia angrily recalls hearing his family who, in his eyes, were trying to minimize his symptoms, saying:

"It's not *that* bad, we too have trouble finding words sometimes . . ."

Another patient whose condition worsened is now rejected and abandoned by his family:

"People don't speak to me as much any more." (J.B.)

Persons with Aphasia and the Health-Care Environment

The hospital milieu is often the first setting for contact between persons with aphasia and others. For many people, the hospital is where the first attempts at communication take place, along with the subsequent awareness of their disability.

"After several attempts at communicating with a volunteer nurse from the Red Cross, I ended up with a pen, a lighter, a watch and a mask. At the time, I couldn't hold a cigarette, and, because of my lack of coordination, I was unable to light the lighter. Time, hours, and minutes, meant nothing to me. Actually, I ended up using the mask to cover my eyes during the nurse's later visits. I was furious at what seemed to me to be an invasion of my world, but I was still unable to express my thoughts." (A.H.)

Another person with aphasia discloses several impressions of doctors' attitudes:

"They always have the same approach: Quick and aloof. I don't get the impression that they are interested in me as an individual, with my own worries. I am a good case. They speak to me as if I were a child, or as if I were drunk: *Mr. A., how's everything? You are looking much better this morning.*" (R.A.)

He adds:

"They aren't friendly. They're distant. They have the cool demeanor of scientists." (R.A.)

This is how he feels during a short examination:

"When they show me a *pen* and I say *hen,* they don't understand. I am unable to do what they want: Perform." (R.A.)

The patient, however, values their competence, but simply wishes they would be more "human":

"They are nonetheless so indispensable to me. I wish that they could communicate more of their knowledge to me. If only they could be friendlier and less hurried."(R.A.)

As one of the most painful memories of the early stages of his illness, one person with aphasia cited the clinical discussions that the medical team held in his presence. He offers this bit of advice:

"You must always presume that the person with aphasia understands a lot more than he appears to." (M.B.)

The same patient, a speech pathologist by profession, offers this plea to people who work or come in contact with persons with aphasia:

"People must be very cautious as to what is said in discussions or in clinical meetings held in the presence of the patient. Negative attitudes can be detected very easily. Always keep in mind that these patients have enough problems without being exposed to the often morbid discussions by medical staff. We all too frequently forget that the patient can hear and understand. It's true that the patient is often unfamiliar with the vocabulary being used, but gestures and other signs are very revealing, especially when the patient is already depressed. We must remember at all times that recovery depends not only on the patient, or the patient's family, but also on the attitudes of the doctors and therapists, who are highly influential." (M.B.)

Another patient defines the ideal attitude towards persons with aphasia. He encourages people not to sympathize, but to empathize with them.

"Perhaps sympathy is "feeling for" someone else, while empathy, is "feeling with" the other person." (C.D.)

The problems faced by persons with aphasia who wish to return to the workplace will be discussed in Chapter 13. Nonetheless, since this chapter features introspective comments, some thoughts on the workforce will be presented here:

"If the person with aphasia is a manual laborer, it seems possible to consider a return to work. Say I work with other people, it would be harder to go back." (L.M.)

This person with aphasia later added:

"At first, people are kind . . . they think of the aphasia. They later become more demanding . . . we, the persons with aphasia get discouraged . . . and we end up quitting." (L.M.)

A person with aphasia who managed to return to work as an orientation counsellor comments that it is difficult for persons with aphasia to differentiate between the aftermath of aphasia and other problems and discomforts that can surface from one day to another.

"I find it hard to distinguish between the actual after-effects of the stroke, and the adjustments to coming back to school after one year of absence." (R.A.)

One theme constantly emerges from these former patients' introspective comments on their linguistic behavior and their psychological and emotional state at the time of the disturbances. That is, persons with aphasia are quite capable of engaging in this type of introspection. Even if these persons present, in varying degrees, a disability affecting communication with others, they are nonetheless individuals with *normal* intellectual capacities, whose thinking processes are, for all intents and purposes, unaffected. This is corroborated by comments in which persons with aphasia compare their illness to *a wall, a prison, or an island*, which cuts them off from the world. These comments also directly attest to the importance of the family and friends as well as the medical team's attitudes.

As for the hospital milieu, the feedback of persons with aphasia reveals that clinical discussions held in their presence greatly disturb them. In these comments, there is the well-founded suggestion that the person's ability to comprehend must never be underestimated. In general, persons with aphasia, like other people with disabilities, hardly appreciate overprotection. Some people even go so far as to use baby talk when addressing the patient! The patients do not want others to speak for them. They would appreciate if people could speak slower and avoid speaking at the same time. If a family member acquires aphasia, the other members should not react abruptly and relieve the victim of all his previous responsibilities. The person with aphasia is still an individual.

These introspective comments also raise a few suggestions (of which this is certainly not an exhaustive list) for speech pathologists or other health-care professionals who are involved in the lengthy rehabilitation process:

- Do not hesitate to use several sensory modes when communicating with persons with aphasia.
- Do not hesitate to solicit the persons' own opinions. Not only are they in the best position for evaluating which aspects of the communication disturbances they would most like to improve through therapy, they can also provide valuable information regarding the most effective treatment strategies.
- Combine gestures and language; use signs and other nonverbal signals to facilitate the person's language comprehension, and to assist the person with linguistic expression.
- Recognize the importance of the therapeutic context, making it as natural as possible.
- Respect the linguistic needs of patients with aphasia by adapting the objectives of therapy to their real needs.

These comments also compel us to consider a problem which has puzzled philosophers from the start; that is, the nature of the relation between thought and language. Several persons with aphasia commented on this problem. For example:

"I tried to analyze what was happening and I wrote: *You would think that the brain is set aside, and not all jumbled.* It seems that the brain is active or passive. Is there a separation between what is active and what isn't? Writing, understanding, drawing, writing . . . Would it be the subject or the idea, even if the idea weren't expressed well? At what point am I thinking, between all forms of expression (drawing, music)?" (M.M.D.)

Indeed, several persons with aphasia have pondered this dilemma. Therefore, although these persons suffer from varying degrees of language impairment, they are still able to think normally. If the patient who stated that: "I no more have the word inside me than I do outside" is telling the truth, then thought must be linked to an internal language that is related to the one which is used in external communication. It is thus tempting, and even dangerous, to presume a non-linguistic dimension to this form of thought. This rash conclusion closely corresponds with the theories of the Russian psychologist A.N. Sokolov[1] who proposed two distinct modes of *thought;* one in the form of an elaborate internal language, similar to the external version, and the other consisting of an internal language reduced to its most basic attributes (predicates). Between these two modes of thought mediation lie many possible intermediary levels. According to Sokolov, the first mode is responsible for the more *complex and arbitrary thoughts,* the second for the concrete thoughts. It therefore follows that although persons with aphasia are incapable of controlling all the thought modes, they do retain the ones required for functioning in everyday life. The presence of aphasia, therefore, significantly damages the relationships between patients and their family. To this effect, aphasia can be considered a "social impairment." To anyone unfamiliar with the condition, persons with aphasia can seem strange. Therefore, these persons' testimonies are informative as well as fascinating.

REFERENCE

1. Sokolov, A.N.: *Inner Speech and Thought*, Plenum, New York, 1972.

CHAPTER 2

AWARENESS OF THE PROBLEM

Y. LEBRUN

ANOSOGNOSIA

At an assembly of the *Société de neurologie* in June 1914, Babinski[7], then head of the neurology clinic at the *Hôpital de la Pitié* in Paris, reported two cases of hemiplegia of the left side accompanied by hypesthesia. Babinski pointed out that during the clinical examination, the two patients showed no sign of confusion or mental deficiency. They were not hallucinating and their speech was coherent. Surprisingly, they did not complain of their hemiplegia; both patients seemed to be oblivious to it. When one of the patients was asked to move her left arm, Babinski claims that she remained "motionless, and did not respond, as if the question had been addressed to someone else." As for the second patient, when asked to move her left arm, she either did nothing or she would simply reply "There. I've done it." Furthermore, one day electrotherapy was suggested. The patient vehemently protested: "But why would I need electrotherapy? I'm not paralyzed!"

Babinski named this obliviousness to one's own hemiplegia "anosognosia."

In the debate that followed Babinski's presentation, Ballet compared the unawareness or denial of hemiplegia to some patients' beliefs that they suffered from no visual deficits, while in fact they were confronted with cortical blindness.

Babinski was the first to draw attention to the obliviousness to motor deficits seen in certain persons with hemiplegia. Fifteen years earlier, Anton[5,6] discovered that some patients suffering from cortical blindness denied having a disability. The work of these two researchers has led to the term "Anton-Babinski Syndrome" occasionally being used synonymously with "anosognosia."

Nine years later, at a meeting of the same society, Barré[8] described a person with hemiplegia who seemed totally unaware of his motor deficit and cried out in disbelief when he was told that the left half of his body was paralyzed. The title of this report was *Etude clinique d'un nouveau cas d'anosognosie de Babinski* (A clinical study of a new case of Babinski's anosognosia).

Since then, the term "anosognosia" has been used to describe cases where patients are neither confused nor mentally disturbed, yet are unaware of their disability despite evident symptoms.

Anosognosia and Language

With Jargon Aphasia

Forty years before Babinski introduced the notion of anosognosia to neurology, Wernicke[35] proposed that patients whose language was paraphasic following a brain lesion were often unaware of their speech problems.

This opinion was echoed by many aphasiologists. Persons with sensory aphasia, in particular the noted "jabberers," are often considered anosognosic. Leischner[28] asserts that such patients are largely unaware of their deficit. Bay[9] concurs and considers that anosognosia is responsible for logorrhea, frequently observed in patients with severe sensory aphasia. Lhermitte and Gautier[29] claim that Wernicke's aphasia is often accompanied by anosognosia. Lecours and Lhermitte[26] differentiated between three types of sensory aphasia. The first type is characterized by "anosognosia which is generally present, and, as a rule, is not absolute." In the second type, "anosognosia is generalized, and may be enduring." Patients suffering from the third type will often be aware of their oral expression problems, but not of impairments in written expression. According to Lecours and Lhermitte, patients suffering from oral deafness are "anosognosic towards errors which slip into their speech."

Some aphasiologists believe that anosognosia is a distinctive feature of jargon aphasia. Alajouanine et al.[4] propose that jargon aphasia stems from an "anosognosic breakdown of the semantic values of language." To Alajouanine and Lhermitte[1], the "anosognosia of jargon aphasics" is obvious. This opinion is shared by Hécaen and Angelergues[15] who note that "the subject is utterly unaware of his jargonaphasia."

Certain specialists, however, do not subscribe to the theory that persons with sensory aphasia—"jabberers"—are unaware of their verbal impairment. Poeck[33] maintains that patients with Wernicke's aphasia are not more oblivious to their deficit than are patients with Broca's aphasia. Hüber et al.[18] also believe that sensory aphasia is not accompanied by anosognosia. Lecours, Travis, and Nespoulous[27] counter that "the anosognosia of Wernicke's aphasia is not so absolute as is generally believed."

Which of these positions is valid? Are persons with sensory aphasia and jargon aphasia aware of their verbal deficits? What is the basis for the widespread opinion that Wernicke's aphasia, especially in severe cases, is often (or invariably) associated with anosognosia?

The idea that persons with sensory aphasia are unaware of their deficit appears to be based largely on the observation that these patients are often loquacious, even logorrheic. If such patients were capable of noticing their abnormal speech production, would they still submit others to meaningless babble? If they could perceive their numerous errors, would they not tend to talk less in order to reduce the likelihood of misunderstandings? Would they not attempt to communicate through alternative nonverbal means?

In a search for answers, clinicians questioned patients themselves. Weinstein et al.[34] asked 18 patients with jargon aphasia whether they suffered from language disturbances. The authors noted that 14 explicitly denied having any difficulty communicating. After interviewing nine patients with sensory aphasia, four with global aphasia and 25 with anomia, Poeck[33] concluded that the patients with sensory aphasia were as aware of their language problem as were the patients with other forms of aphasia.

The conflicts within these findings are undoubtedly linked to the difficulty in accurately interpreting the verbal responses of patients with Wernicke's aphasia to questions pertaining to their condition and their awareness thereof. Since these patients generally suffer from severe comprehension deficits, it is impossible to ascertain whether or not the patients adequately understand the questions. Their deviant use of language means that the interpretation of these patients' responses remains conjectural.

Consequently, patients themselves cannot serve as reliable sources of information as long as they are suffering from sensory aphasia. It seems that only people who have recovered their verbal capacities can provide valid data. This situation is exemplified in cases of paroxysmic aphasia, a transitory form which subsides along with the epileptic seizure that induced it.

Lecours and Joanette[25] studied a patient with this syndrome. During the seizures, the patient suffered from predominantly sensory aphasia. Between seizures, the patient regained his verbal skills and could intelligibly describe what he had experienced during the paroxysmal phase. The patient explained that, at the time, he was aware of experiencing language problems. He noticed that he could not understand what people said to him, and that he was unable to speak properly. He could not, however, determine what was deficient in his verbal production. In other words, he knew he was making mistakes in his performance, but he did not know the precise nature of the errors. He was unaware that his paroxysmal jargon was often interspersed with English expressions, yet his mother tongue and working language was French. He was totally unaware that "tuware," a neologism, frequently appeared in his jabbering, sometimes with minor phonemic variations. He did know, however, that at the end of the seizure he tended to recover the ability to write legibly before being able to speak clearly. When he needed to communicate verbally during the terminal phase of a paroxysmal seizure, he would usually resort to writing.

These observations support the findings of Alajouanine and Sabouraud[3] who also describe a case of paroxysmal aphasia. During the seizures, the patient knew that she could not speak properly, but was unable to detect her mistakes: "I realize that it (what I say) isn't right, because people are laughing, but I can't hear it; I don't know what I'm saying."

Recurring Utterances

Whereas in the cases studied by Lecours and Joanette[25] and Alajouanine and Sabouraud[3] the patients displayed some awareness of their disability, the patient observed by Lebrun and Leleux[23] appeared to exhibit a total anosognosia regarding his language deficit. Upon emerging from a coma induced by a head injury, the patient displayed severe comprehension problems. In addition, the patient emitted a recurring utterance: No matter what he intended to say, the only syllable uttered was "TAN." He would generally repeat this syllable several times in succession, like the well-known case described by Broca[11].

A few weeks later, the neurolinguistic condition of the patient improved. The comprehension problems abated and the recurring utterances gave way to intelligible yet occasionally paraphasic oral performance.

Since the patient was once again capable of verbal communication, he was asked if, during his aphasic state, he realized that he was always uttering the same syllable—"tan." The patient was very surprised to learn that he was suffering from this particular type of aphasia upon recovering from his coma. He had absolutely no recollection of that experience! Yet his behavior was not that of someone suffering from retroactive amnesia induced by a head injury. The patient did recall a series of events (treatments, visits, etc..) that took place in the days following his coma. It was only his stereotypical verbal behavior which left no imprint in his memory. There can be no denying that in this case, the patient experienced anosognosia at the time of his stereotypical aphasia.

These examples demonstrate that patients with Wernicke's aphasia or recurring utterances may possess little or, in some cases, no awareness of their verbal disturbances.

The Mechanisms at Work

In an attempt to account for this obliviousness that certain patients display towards their verbal deficits, the following section will examine possible explanations for anosognosia.

Verbal Deafness

There may be reason to believe that the verbal comprehension difficulties which characterize sensory aphasia account for the obliviousness of patients to the inadequacy of their verbal performance. Can subjects who can no longer correctly decipher linguistic messages evaluate the correctness of what they themselves say or write? To assess the quality of one's verbal performance, is it not necessary to understand for yourself the way one understands others? It seems that persons who experience difficulties decoding can no longer easily compare what they perceive orally or visually with the knowledge they have of language. The patients will realize that they can no longer assess their performance, but will be unable to identify their errors. This seems to have been the case with the subjects studied by Lecours and Joanette[25] and by Alajouanine and Sabouraud[3].

Auditory Feedback

Clearly, the explanation above cannot account for the anosognosia which seemed to be in evidence in the case reported by Lebrun and Leleux[23]. Indeed, it is not necessary to understand what one said to perceive that one is constantly repeating the same syllable. Moreover, a listener can diagnose a case of recurring utterances without knowledge of the patient's mother tongue. Even a patient with severe comprehension disturbances should still be able to note such aberrant production. Therefore verbal deafness cannot possibly account for the patients' unawareness of their stereotypical verbal behavior. What, then, could explain anosognosia in patients manifesting recurring utterances?

It is possible that some persons with aphasia are no longer able to listen and speak at the same time; they subsequently cannot hear what they are saying while they are talking. Patients with aphasia have already confirmed that a lesion in the brain can impair one's ability to perform two tasks simultaneously. Wulf[36] could no longer do two things simultaneously once she acquired aphasia. Hall[14], another person with aphasia, notes that a patient suffering from motor aphasia and hemiplegia may be totally unable to understand speech when he is walking on uneven ground, but will comprehend normally if not distracted. De Morsier[12] described a person with aphasia who normally did not suffer from dysphagia, but if she was spoken to during her meal, would swallow the wrong way. She could not eat and understand at the same time. Wulf[36] experienced difficulties with speaking during meals and with understanding texts when asked to read aloud.

Normally, the speaker is both the sender and the receiver, speaking and monitoring the output at the same time. This dual task may become impossible for the person with aphasia. Moss[32] reported that at the onset of his aphasia, he was unable to express himself verbally while simultaneously monitoring the accuracy of his speech.

Therefore, it is quite possible that, for certain persons with aphasia, auditory feedback is interrupted because speech production cannot occur in conjunction with speech perception. The patient subsequently becomes functionally deaf to what he is saying as soon as he begins speaking.

This theory regarding the interruption of auditory feedback can explain two types of observations. Alajouanine et al.[2], noticed that the speech of subjects suffering from jargon aphasia was not at all affected when their auditory feedback was electronically delayed; a process which generally disorients normal speakers. Boller's[10] research corroborates these findings.

Secondly, Alajouanine and Lhermitte[1] observed that certain patients with jargon aphasia apparently recognize the inadequacy of their verbal output if they hear a recording of their speech. "If they are made to listen to their own words recorded on tape," the authors note, "they are amazed; they laugh it off or they become angry because they feel that others are taking them for fools . . ."

When patients with jargon aphasia listen to a recording of their speech, they are only listeners. It is perhaps the singularity of this task that allows them to recognize the deviance of their verbal performance, something of which they were unaware at the time they were speaking.

Self Image

"Jabberers," in contrast, do not find fault with their verbal performance when they listen to it later. Zangwill[37] and Kinsbourne and Warrington[20] noted, in fact, that these patients seem to accept a recording of their speech, but exclaim in surprise when they hear their utterances repeated by a third person. Likewise, they feel that their written expression is adequate, but reject identical texts written by someone else.

What can account for this behavioral difference? Can it be that upon hearing or seeing their production the patients perceive, but refuse to acknowledge, the inadequacies so as not to harm their self image? Are they trying to dispel any suspicions as to their disability? Is it possible that they act as if they were in full control of their language capacities in order to sustain the belief that they are still eminently verbal? Testimonies by persons with aphasia have illustrated the extent to which the loss of language can affect a person's self perception. Wulf[36] notes that aphasia can be a devastating blow to the self esteem. Van Veen (in a work by Heylen[17]) reports that he was unable to accept the fact that he had aphasia. Moss[31] also found it difficult not being as articulate as before.

It is therefore possible that, in some cases, patients are aware of the inadequacy of their verbal production, but choose to ignore it in order to protect their self image.

The Phatic Function of Language

In all likelihood, the need to retain the self image of a *Homo loquens* is not the only reason that some patients seemingly ignore their verbal deficits. Perhaps some patients with aphasia know that their speech is unintelligible, but they speak nonetheless, in order not to sink into a desperate silence and subsequently eliminate any potential contact with family and friends.

Speech has other functions beyond the transmission of information. Indeed, it acts as a link between the speaker and the listener. For people in close relationships, the prime use of speech is to maintain and reinforce intimacy and attachment. Speech is a unifying force, regardless of the semantic content of the message. People discuss a wide range of topics, solely to foster the feelings of belonging and togetherness. Speech, in this case, plays a phatic rather than an informative role.

Perhaps certain persons with aphasia continue to speak because their speech, although it may be too deviant or recurrent to be informative, still retains its phatic quality. If the patients were to remain silent, they would founder in loneliness, lose contact with family and friends, and would no longer feel close to loved ones. Even if their speech is devoid of informative value, at least it can still be used to achieve contact. Even if the patients are understood poorly, or not at all, the verbal exchange allows for a transmission of human warmth which cannot be achieved in silence.

Dashed Hopes

Another possibility is that some patients who emit recurring utterances continue to speak because, with each fresh attempt at verbal expression, they believe that 'this time, at last, the words will come out the way I want.' This hope may be fueled by an occasional non-recurring or even acceptable verbal utterance. In fact, especially when in emotional states[24], most of these patients do occasionally produce a correct word or short phrase. Perhaps these intermittent "verbal ejaculations" foster hopes, inevitably dashed, that the deviance will disappear with the next performance.

Hughlings Jackson[19] proposed that recurring utterances did not originate from the injured area of the brain, but rather from a subordinate center of the nervous system that can no longer be controlled by the damaged area. If so, we can assume that the patient, when he wants to talk, activates the part of his brain that selects the correct words. Before externalization, however, these words are first transmitted to a subsidiary center, where they are not processed properly. They become blocked, and only recurring utterances are produced. The patient can be said to have been cheated, at the last minute, by an execution function which defies the production and control mechanisms in the brain.

ANOSODIAPHORIA

In his message to the *Société de neurologie* in 1914, Babinski[7] proposed that certain persons with hemiplegia "while not ignoring their paralysis, did not seem to attach any importance to it." He suggested that the term 'anosodiaphoria' be used to refer to the indifference that certain patients exhibit towards their disability.

Like anosognosia, anosodiaphoria is not limited to motor deficits. It can also be observed with respect to intellectual disturbances, as seen in the now classic case described by Liepmann[30] early in this century. A right-handed patient, when asked to perform a task with one hand, spontaneously used his right hand and, most often, did not execute the task properly. If, moments later, without the request being repeated, the patient was merely asked to perform the same task with his left hand, he was able to comply satisfactorily, proving that he had understood and remembered the command. Why, then, did he not attempt to improve the performance of his right hand? Why was he content with a right-hand performance that did not correspond with the clearly understood task? Why, Liepmann pertinently noted, was the patient satisfied with the inadequate performance of his right hand, and why was there no self-correction? Finally, and most importantly, why, given the apraxia in his right hand, did he not spontaneously use his left hand, whose performance was considerably superior?

Apparently the patient was indifferent to and unaffected by the performance of his right hand. In other words, he was anosodiaphoric to his apraxia.

Anosodiaphoria is observable in patients with aphasia as well. Perhaps some patients are aware of the inadequacy of their language production, but are indifferent to it. These patients may speak because they want (or need) to speak, but they are not concerned with their errors. The quality of their verbal performance is of no importance to them. The communication disorder is accepted as was apraxia in the case reported by Liepmann.

The theory that certain persons with aphasia are anosodiaphoric towards their verbal deficit could explain logorrhea. As a result of the lesion, the patient becomes talkative and derives extreme pleasure from speaking, but is totally unconcerned with the effects of his babble. He is oblivious to the deviant nature of his performance, and succumbs to his intense and unbounded desire to speak.

In such cases, the anosodiaphoria is limited to communication problems. Anosodiaphoria may also be more generalized. For example, after a head injury or severe stroke, patients may be indifferent to their condition. The head trauma may be so severe that the shock virtually anesthetizes them. The patients float in a 'no man's land' between life and death, unable to understand or to react to what is happening to them. They are apparently oblivious to the deficits induced by the lesion. Moss[31], although he was aware of having aphasia and alexia at the onset of his illness, was not distressed at the thought of being unable to communicate verbally. He was also nonchalant about the consequences that his aphasia would inevitably have on his family and professional life. At the onset of her condition, Wulf[36] also experienced detachment. She felt as if she were in a "care-free limbo" and nothing could harm her. The French doctor who described his aphasia in *Documenta Geigy* of 1969, experienced this same sensation: "I was utterly indifferent; as anxious and distressed as I generally was before my illness, now I was just as detached from my surroundings."

George Simenon, in his novel *Les anneaux de Bicêtre*, describes the initial anosodiaphoria of certain persons with aphasia. His protagonist, René Maugras, suddenly acquires aphasia following a stroke, but he is absolutely unconcerned by his condition. Simenon wrote, "His **disability** is pleasant enough, it's somehow as if he weren't anybody any more . . . he has no more problems, responsibilities. He was never so carefree in all his life."

When it does surface, this initial indifference is usually short-lived. With time, the patient emerges from the cocoon induced by the brain injury. Little by little, the patient becomes aware of the severity of the condition, and realizes the extent of his disability. This realization may cause the initial indifference to give way to subsequent dysphoria.

DYSPHORIA

Dysphoria is a psychological condition characterized by deep sadness, profound discouragement, and intense anxiety. The person with dysphoria is defeated, hopeless, or terribly worried.

Dysphoria may surface when the person with aphasia, after an initial indifference phase, begins to appreciate the severity of his condition. Sometimes this painful realization is hastened, even brought on, by the attending medical staff. Under a verbal examination, the patient with aphasia may suddenly notice a deficit which had previously escaped his detection. Difficulties in complying with linguistic exercises often expose patients to the extent of their disability. This brutal revelation can lead to extreme dejection. It is essential that health-care professionals keep this eventuality in mind when testing patients shortly after the onset of aphasia.

In addition to discouragement brought on by the awareness of the verbal deficit, patients who acquire post-stroke aphasia may be very anxious that the stroke may recur and aggravate the already acute problems. This fear may become an obsession, with patients living in constant fear that their condition may deteriorate. The traumatic awareness of the illness is thus compounded by fears of potential deterioration.

Even if patients are not obsessed by fears that the aphasia may aggravate, they may still become quite discouraged due to profound feelings of diminishment. They feel as if aphasia has deprived them of a typically human quality, branding them "inferior." It is surely this painful sense of worthlessness that the novelist Valéry Larbaud attempted to convey when, suffering from a severe case of aphasia, he would reply "déchu, déchu" (fallen, fallen) to friends who inquired as to his condition (Lebrun[21]).

Although patients may not be in perpetual misery over the verbal impotence brought on by aphasia, the inability to communicate can be, on occasion, extremely painful for the patient. Caroline Aupick, Charles Beaudelaire's mother, reported occasional desperate episodes experienced by her son, who had aphasia, when people didn't understand what he was trying to communicate by means of the recurring utterance: "Cre nom nom." In a letter to a friend, Aupick relates,

> "His book of poems (the anthology *Les Epaves*) often induced terrible outbursts of rage. He would have something to tell me about the book, and I just couldn't understand. Recently, picking up this miserable book, he thrust it in my face until I had to step back; he then became absolutely furious because I couldn't understand, and stamped his foot with all his might. Finally, exhausted, he threw himself upon the couch and, minutes later, yelled at the top of his lungs, waving his legs in the air and howling like a beast."[22]

These catastrophic reactions are not uncommon in persons with aphasia who, like Larbaud and Baudelaire, are still able to understand language fairly well, but find it exceedingly difficult to express themselves. Aware of their inability to communicate verbally, the patients founder in despair. If these feelings do not subside, the extreme hopelessness can degenerate into chronic depression or negativism.

Even a person with a moderate case of aphasia that does not fully impair verbal expression may become discouraged. Verbal aptitudes are such an essential aspect of human nature that even their partial loss may be hard to accept. Self-acceptance, following the post-aphasia transformations, may be difficult to achieve. As seen above, it seems that some patients with aphasia react by denying their deficit, as if they were still as verbal as before the illness. Others, on the contrary, are aware of their verbal deficiency, and are subsequently distressed. Although they are fully aware of the change, they cannot accept it. Dysphoria is thus a direct result of neither being able to hide from the disability, nor to accept it.

IMPACT ON LANGUAGE RE-EDUCATION

Should the emotional state of patients with aphasia, and their awareness of the problem, be taken into consideration by the speech pathologist who treats them? Evidently, yes.

In fact, speech therapy risks being fruitless if the patient is profoundly discouraged. The feelings of impotence and uselessness that beset the patients sap the self-assurance and motivation which they need to benefit from therapy. A certain amount of enthusiasm is required to regain, even partially, verbal skills.

If the patients wallow in self pity or utterly reject their new condition, they will be unprepared to begin rehabilitation. At this stage, effective treatment of aphasia should be two-pronged. It should aim not only to increase the verbal capacities of the patient, but should also encourage the patient to accept a condition that differs from the one prior to the illness, i.e., a less flattering self image than before. If this acceptance does not come about, internal conflicts can induce depression and negativism.

Of course this does not imply that patients should be encouraged to resign themselves to their fate. On the contrary, therapy should constantly strive to assist patients in improving their performance, to outdo themselves. While stimulating the patients' progress, therapy should also, it is believed, ensure that patients do not renounce their new condition. Without self-acceptance, patients run a strong risk of gaining nothing from therapy.

Is the situation more favorable in cases where patients seem to be unaware of the problem and are subsequently not bothered by it? Apparently not. In fact, many therapists consider anosognosia a hindrance to the patients' progress and that this syndrome should be eliminated as soon as possible if the therapy is to be effective. If patients believe that they are expressing themselves properly, or at least intelligibly, it is more difficult to expect correction than if they recognize their speech errors. This is why it is important that at the start of therapy patients be aware of the aberrant nature of their utterances. In some cases it is admittedly difficult to inform the patients that their speech is not intelligible. This is particularly true in cases of recurring utterances.

What reaction is called for when patients are unaware that with each attempt at speech, they utter the same syllable? Ducarne de Ribaucourt[(13)] recommends that the therapist imitate the verbal behavior of the patient, but with dramatic exaggeration. Helm-Estabrooks et al.[(16)] ostensibly write the patient's recurring utterance on a piece of paper and hold it before the patient each time he emits, or is about to emit, the utterance. Another means of helping patients become aware of their verbal output is through sound and video recordings of their speech. The actual strategy used is of less importance than the need to make the patient aware of the verbal behavior to be modified.

It appears, therefore, that the awareness of the problem, and the patient's emotional reaction to this knowledge, are significant elements in the clinical description of patients with aphasia. Patients' ideas about and reactions towards their deficit affect their behavior as well as their morale. In order to assess the patient fully and to maximize the effectiveness of therapy, specialists must be vigilant for signs of anosognosia, anosodiaphoria, and reactional dysphoria.

REFERENCES

1. Alajouanine, T. & F. Lhermitte: Des anosognosies électives. *Encéphale,* **46**: 505–519, 1957.
2. Alajouanine, T. et al.: Les composantes phonémiques et sémantiques de la jargonaphasie. *Revue Neurologique (Paris),* **110**: 5–20, 1964.
3. Alajouanine, T. & O. Sabouraud: Les perturbations paroxystiques du langage dans l'épilepsie, *Encéphale,* **49**: 95–133, 1960.
4. Alajouanine, T., O. Sabouraud & B. de Ribaucourt: Le jargon des aphasiques. *Journal de Psychologie Normale et Pathologique,* **45**: 158–180, 293–329, 1952.
5. Anton, G.: Uber Herderkrankungen des Gehirns, welche vom Patienten selbst nicht wahrgenommen werden. *Wiener klinische Wochenschrift,* **11**: 227–229, 1898.
6. Anton, G.: Uber die Selbstwahrnehmungen der Herderkrankungen des Gehirns durch den Kranken bei Rindenblindheit und Rindentaubheit. *Archiv für Psychiatrie und Nervenkrankheiten,* **32**: 86–127, 1899.
7. Babinski, J.: Contribution à l'étude des troubles mentaux dans l'hémipléglie organique cérébrale (Anosognosie). *Revue Neurologique (Paris),* **27**: 845–847, 1914.
8. Barré, J., L. Morin & Kaiser: Étude clinique d'un nouveau cas d'anosognosie de Babinski. *Revue Neurologique (Paris)* **36**: 500–502, 1923.
9. Bay, E.: Principles of classification and their influence on our concepts of aphasia, **in** *Disorders of Language,* De Reuck, A. & M. O'Connor (eds). Churchill, London, 1964.
10. Boller, F.: Delayed auditory feedback: A possible clue to the mechanism of some types of aphasia, **in** *Problems of Aphasia.* Lebrun, Y., & R. Hoops (eds). Swets and Zeitlinger, Lisse, 1979.
11. Broca, P.: Remarques sur le siège de la faculté de langage suivies d'une observation d'aphémie. *Bulletin de la Société d'Anatomie,* **6**: 330–357, 1861.
12. De Morsier, G.: Les troubles de la déglutition et des mouvements de la langue dans l'anarthrie (aphasie motrice). *Practica Oto-Rhino-Laryngologica,* **11**: 125–133, 1949.
13. Ducarne de Ribaucourt, B.: *Rééducation sémiologique de l'aphasie,* Masson, Paris, 1986.
14. Hall, A.: Return from Silence, A Personal Experience. *Journal of Speech and Hearing Disorders,* **26**: 174–177, 1961.
15. Hécaen, H. & R. Angelergues: *Pathologie du langage,* Larousse, Paris, 1965.
16. Helm-Estabrooks, N., P. Emery & M. Albert: Treatment of Aphasic Perseveration (TAP) program. *Archives of Neurology,* **44**: 1253–1255, 1987.
17. Heylen, L.: *Het Woord ligt me op de tong,* Acco, Leuven, 1982.
18. Hüber, W. et al.: Die Wernicke-Aphasie. *J Neurol,* **210**: 77–97, 1975.
19. Hughlings Jackson, J.: On Affections of Speech from Disease of the Brain. *Brain,* **2**: 203–220. 1880.
20. Kinsbourne, M. & E. Warrington: Jargon aphasia. *Neuropsychologica,* **1**: 27–37, 1963.
21. Lebrun, Y.: The Inside of Aphasia, **in** *The Management of Aphasia.* Lebrun, Y. & R. Hoops (eds). Swets and Zeitlinger, Lisse, 1978.

22. Lebrun, Y. et al.: L'aphasie de Charles Beaudelaire. *Revue Neurologique (Paris),* **125**: 310–316, 1971.
23. Lebrun, Y. & C. Leleux: Anosognosie et aphasie. *Archives Suisses de Neurologie, Neurochirurgie et de Psychiatrie,* **130**: 25–38, 1982.
24. Lebrun, Y.: Aphasia with Recurrent Alterance: A Review. *British Journal of Disorders of Communication,* **21**: 3–10, 1986.
25. Lecours, A.R. & Y. Joanette: Linguistic and other psychological aspects of paroxysmal aphasia. *Brain & Language,* **10**: 1–23, 1980.
26. Lecours, A.R. & F. Lhermitte: *L'aphasie,* Flammarion, Paris, 1979.
27. Lecours, A.R., L. Travis & J.-L. Nespoulous: Néologismes et anosognosie. *Grammatica 7,* **1**: 101–114, (Université de Toulouse-Le Mirail),1980.
28. Leischner, A.: *Aphasien und Sprachentwicklungsstörungen,* Thieme, Stuttgart, 1979.
29. Lhermitte, F. & J. Gautier: Aphasia, **in** Vinken, P. & G. Bruyn (eds). *Handbook of Clinical Neurology,* **4**: 84–104, 1969.
30. Liepmann, H.: Das Krankheitsbild der Apraxie (Motorische Asymbolie). *Monatsschrift für Psychiatrie und Neurologie,* **8**: 15–44, 102–132, 182–197, 1900.
31. Moss, S.:*Recovery With Aphasia,* University of Illinois Press, Urbana, 1972.
32. Moss, S.: Notes from an aphasiologist, or different strokes for different folks, **in** *Recovery in Aphasics.* Lebrun, Y. & R. Hoops (eds). Swets and Zeitlinger, Lisse, 1976.
33. Poeck, K.: Stimmung und Krankheitseinsicht bei Aphasien. *Archiv für Psychiatrie und Nervenkrankeiten,* **216**: 246–254, 1972.
34. Weinstein, E. et al.: Meaning in Jargon Aphasia. *Cortex,* **2**: 155–187, 1966.
35. Wernicke, C.: *Der aphasische Symptomencomplex,* Cohn & Weigert, Breslau, 1874.
36. Wulf, H.: *Aphasia, My World Alone,* Wayne University Press, Detroit, 1973.
37. Zangwill, O.: *Disorders of Language.* De Reuck, A. & M. O'Connor (eds). Churchill, London, 1964.

CHAPTER 3

THE PHYSICAL EXPERIENCE OF THE PERSON WITH APHASIA

J. METELLUS, V. LEFEBVRE-DES-NOETTES-GISQUET, AND I. VENDEUVRE

The aim of this chapter is not to substitute words for reality, for a pathology. The physical symptoms which result from lesions in the right and left hemispheres are well known and need not be listed here. Regardless of whether aphasia occurs, the lesions are manifested by distinct symptoms and are always directly responsible for physical disabilities that complicate organic hemiplegia. It is the way in which the illness is expressed that will vary according to whether or not the patient can speak. Observations by several authors will clarify certain aspects of this topic.

THE BODILY EXPRESSION OF PERSONS WITH APHASIA

Beginning with Froment, efforts to evaluate the reactions of persons with aphasia towards their motor deficits have been fairly successful. Patients invariably experience humiliation coupled with discouragement.

Alajouanine[2] reports that Valéry Larbaud retained his pleasant nature and charming smile:

> "He willingly participated in the rehabilitation exercises which many persons with aphasia find infuriating. He seemed to consider them a game (in fact tailored as much as possible to his tastes, such as the blank map of the Bourbonnais region used to jog the memory of familiar places). His tolerance of the symptoms of his illness did not extend to his right hemiplegia which, especially in the early stages, was a constant source of distress. The ill-received physical rehabilitation techniques ultimately had to be abandoned.
>
> "A few years later the situation changed; Larbaud had recovered his former reserve and was a portrait of resignation with melancholic overtones. He tended to withdraw in silence, only listening to the radio or consulting a dictionary. Some days he refused visitors; perhaps out of shame, but also out of the need for seclusion. Maurice Constantin-Weyer, a relative, reported that one day he met Larbaud in the streets of Vichy, where he was being taken on an outing. 'Déchu, déchu' (fallen, fallen) Larbaud cried, shaking his head sadly."

Larbaud, like all persons with aphasia, was evidently troubled by his motor deficit.

A PILOT'S SUCCESSFUL REINTEGRATION

Similarities can be observed in the case of the pilot with aphasia studied by Jules Froment[3]. This man suffered at age 30 from right hemiplegia accompanied by aphasia. He partially recovered the use of his right arm, yet his spastic right hand was virtually ineffectual. Over a year after the stroke, the pilot was advised to retrain because it was believed that he would not be able to tolerate the constant physical strain inherent in aerial exercises. His superiors also feared that his reflexes were impaired and that he would be less capable of responding to unforeseen events.

Sergeant R. could not accept this verdict and asked to be put to the test. His superiors told him to fly to 10,000 feet, then 15,000, then 20,000. On the basis of his fine performance, he was allowed to return to work. After an adjustment period of a few months, Sergeant R. was once again flying as an air gunner, as well as working in the particularly demanding position of location photographer. Shortly afterwards, he continued to work at the base, where he participated fully in all the regular activities.

Despite his disability, he manipulated the guns, not an easy task in flight, with a precision which allowed him to achieve a performance comparable to that of his colleagues. In addition, he continued to take oblique pictures with a hand-held camera weighing close to 30 pounds. Few of his colleagues were able to obtain pictures that were as fine and as well-centered, even with the use of both hands. The pilot had developed a technique which allowed him to snap pictures using his healthy hand while simultaneously positioning the camera as it lay on his other arm.

The pilot's successful adaptation and mastery over his disabilities is proof of his extraordinary mental acuity. Two years after the stroke, Sergeant R. was appointed to the photography division where he performed extremely complex maneuvers: daytime flights at 18,000 feet, with only one other pilot, the shooting of nearly 1,000 photographs, and developing negatives at night. He was also responsible for the arduous task of identifying prints on a map and preparing photographic frames, without blurring a single one. All this was accomplished without the use of his right hand. He occasionally undertook an additional afternoon flight as well. The pilot willingly continued in this manner for between one and a half to two months. R. was subsequently congratulated by the minister for winning first prize among the four crews responsible for that mission.

Exactly two years after the stroke, R. participated in the intelligence aviation championships. The featured events were shooting, bombing, photography, and artillery manipulation. Sergeant R. won that year, as well as in the three subsequent annual championships.

Eight years later, during the war, he piloted on reconnaissance flights and bombings, where he showcased his talent as well as his technical proficiency. He consequently earned this commendation from the division: "Ever since the hostilities began, this elite air gunner with remarkable drive and professional commitment executed several in-depth reconnaissance missions at night and bombings during the day.

Two missions were hampered by violent winds and an attack by anti-aircraft missiles, yet they were brilliantly executed nonetheless."

In this case, the physical disability did not affect the war-time performance of this pilot; he continually displayed physical courage and determination.

Captain X., with whom R. had often co-piloted, claims that R. never appeared to be intellectually deficient and that he quickly mastered the operation of new aircraft which were little understood by other servicemen. Captain X. attests that among the NCOs and his squadron-mates, R. was considered influential. He also believed R. to be well balanced and extremely cool-headed, even during tiring missions; moreover, he exhibited normal intellectual abilities.

Throughout the patient's account of his illness and his disability, he reflected upon the lack of understanding of those around him. He realized that at the onset of his illness his superiors had little confidence in him; some felt that he was "crazy." All persons with hemiplegia undergo similar experiences, but this pilot could not easily convey the idea that he could still work as well as before. The patient, however, was quite capable of clearly narrating his eventful life-story.

Well-respected by all his superiors, R. endured all the hazards and unforeseen circumstances that characterize his profession; in peace time, when he executed reconnaissance missions, and during the war, when he embarked upon dangerous attack missions. Although his superiors were convinced of his psychological abilities and adaptive skills, R. remained unsatisfied with his achievements.

In cases where persons were formerly eloquent and spoke without stumbling or hesitating before they acquired aphasia, a concomitant physical disability, especially right hemiplegia, will consequently disturb their psyche as well as their speech. Dysarthria, logorrhea, or word-finding problems may also surface. One can only hope that there are "luckier" people, whose professional abilities are not only unaffected but are clearly enhanced following the brain injury. The following case illustrates another such scenario.

THE FLOURISHING PAINTER

This person was perhaps more content than the previous subject. A painter with word-finding difficulties, whose logorrhea was replete with nominal and verbal paraphasias, was able to pursue his career thanks to the dexterity of his upper right limb. According to connoisseurs, this painter experienced an increase in visual acuity, especially in terms of color, outline, and general creativity.

Alajouanine describes his patient in the following manner: "It seems that our painter's artistic production goes on as if nothing had happened, and that in him the aphasic and the artist live together on two distinct planes. He himself will admit this when he is congratulated upon his artistic activity. 'There are in me two men, the one who paints, who is normal while he is painting, and the other one who is lost in the mist, who does not stick to life . . . I am saying very poorly what I mean . . . There are inside me the one who grasps reality, life; there is the other who is lost as regards abstract thinking. When I am painting, I am outside my own life; my way of seeing things is even sharper than before. I find everything again, I am a whole man. Even my right hand, that seems strange to me, I do not notice when I am painting. There are two men: one who is compelled by reality to paint, and the other one, the fool who cannot manage words any more'.[1] Is it possible to describe better than our painter, despite his faulty speech, the discrepancy he felt within himself between his speech abilities and expression through his representative art?".[(1)]

THE OBLIGATORY USE OF THE UNAFFECTED HALF OF THE BODY

Most persons with aphasia whose professions require the use of the right upper limb (for example Larbaud, Beaudelaire, or the pilot treated by Froment) find themselves unable to use their right hands.

Maurice Ravel

Alajouanine[(1)] had this to say regarding the pianist and composer, Ravel:

> "Piano playing is very difficult since, in addition to difficulty in reading, this patient with aphasia has to search for the location of notes on the keyboard. He sometimes misplaces notes without being aware of it. For instance he plays the mi-mi instead of do-do arpeggio, and plays it again and again, until his fingers are placed on the proper keys.
>
> "He plays scales quite well, both major and minor ones. Dieses [sharps] and flats are well marked. There is just a praxic difficulty. He can play with only one hand (the right one) the beginning of *Ma Mère l'Oye.* With both hands he cannot decipher. He needs many exercises to play in that way. In spite of numerous exercises during a whole week he cannot succeed in playing the be-

---

[1]Alajouanine, T. "Aphasia and Artistic Realization" in, Martha Taylor Sarno, (ed.), *Aphasia: Selected Readings.* New York: Appleton Century Crofts, p. 236, 1972.

ginning of *Pavane*, even with separate hands. On the contrary, he has a greater performance ability when he plays by heart pieces of his own composition. He suddenly gives a right idea of the beginning of *Tombeau de Couperin,* an extremely rapid and difficult passage. Seven or eight bars are played almost perfectly, and he plays them, transposing to the lower [third], without any error. When attempting an unknown piece he finds a much greater difficulty; he cannot play more than two or three notes of a piece by Scarlatti which he did not previously know.

> "Musical notation is very difficult, although better preserved than plain writing. He writes dictated notes slowly and with numerous errors, but copying is almost impossible and requires from the patient enormous effort. In contrast, writing by heart a portion of his *Entretiens de la Belle et de la Bête,* though difficult and slow, is performed better than the other tasks. Notes are better and more quickly placed, and he seems mainly disturbed by writing apraxia."

In some patients, the physical deficits go hand in hand with the inability to read, write, and give instructions — a phenomenon which is particularly disturbing for, say, a conductor. These patients lose some of their sense of rhythm, which normally allows for downstrokes and upstrokes in writing, annotating texts, and drawing. When aphasia is coupled with right hemiplegia, the patient's psyche is rendered even more fragile and vulnerable. He usually learns to remain silent, to express himself with gestures. At best he will come to accept this condition, if the situation is not aggravated by the loss of the ability to communicate through gestures.

Many persons with aphasia and hemiplegia consider this condition intolerable. To quote Mrs. B. "No talking, no moving — I want to die." A Sister of Charity confided "the most humiliating thing is being washed." In fact, these patients often convey their distress over their daily experiences through cries or moans, their only means of expression when they can no longer command language and their bodies.

Sabadel

This case was published by Philippe Van Eeckhout along with professors François Lhermitte and Jean-Louis Signoret. The artist Sabadel was rehabilitated at the Salpêtrière Hospital by Van Eeckhout[7] (see Chapter 5) who wrote:

> "Although Sabadel is no longer optimistic about recovering the use of his right hand, he evidently does not believe either that he will be able to express himself fully by using his left hand. He is

quite willing to use his left hand in therapy but not beyond that context. This explains the absence of effort to attempt to recover, with his left hand, what the illness deprived him of his professional and social life. For the patient, drawing has not re-assumed its role as a creative medium; it is simply a means of communicating with the outside world."

"In order for Sabadel to find himself again — and also for him to become aware of the possibilities which are still within his reach — we must find another solution. Subsequently we asked him one day to describe a day in his life. The daily activities were meticulously and humorously related. His family life appeared to be well-adjusted. Sabadel's place was particularly evident, for example, in depictions of interaction with the whole family, solitary activities such as painting or drawing, re-education exercises, fixing the children's snack, preparing the table for supper, and greeting his wife upon her return. Evidently, a new equilibrium had been attained within the Sabadel family, largely thanks to the tireless efforts and the responsible character of the patient's wife. By observing this comic strip, where everything seems to be slightly more than perfect, one can surmise that our patient is not at all troubled by his condition, and that he is suffering from neither motor nor linguistic disturbances.

"To confirm our theories, we asked Sabadel to try to imagine how others saw him. We proposed the following exercise: How does he feel judged by society? His response was a draw-ing that reflected, in part, the indifference that he senses emanates from people when he is in Paris. The other element in the drawing is the curiosity displayed by the inhabitants of his native village. The only thing missing was his view of the working world. He chiefly describes himself and his disabilities. He humorously related how he no longer sees things in the same way as those around him. From this we concluded that he is aware of his professional inadequacy. He justifies this observation by saying that other people are victims of the modern harried lifestyle."

"At any rate, Sabadel will not spontaneously triumph over his limitations. He lacks the energy required to recover on his own. Rehabilitation is not advancing. It lacks vitality. The therapist feels as if he has reached an impasse. After having covered so much ground, it would be pointless to stop then and there. But how could they get the ball rolling again? The inspiration came from a television program on literature. The guest authors volunteered to recount their life stories before an audience of thousands. Why could Sabadel not do the same? Perhaps he could speak for all persons with aphasia and describe what he had felt and experienced from the day that he emerged from his coma.

"As it happened, when Sabadel sat before us, it was as if we were sitting around the bargaining table: 'We can no longer do much for you; your treatment will end — unless you accept to go public with your account of your illness. Draw it, we will give you fifteen days to do it. Your future depends on it'.

"We added offhand that the 'book' that he is encouraged to produce may represent a 'Trojan Horse' on a professional scale. Sabadel listened to us, astonished. He was surprised by our tone of voice, and by this seemingly intentional 'blackmail.' He was reticent at first, but finally accepted, still fairly unconvinced.

"We already mentioned that persons with aphasia suffer as much from being considered different from before as from their inability to speak. Nonetheless, in this case, Sabadel was able to continue to express himself through drawings[6]. Better yet, he could create, proving that expression and creativity are not limited to speech. This is true not only for musicians, sculptors, and painters, but also for those who can express themselves with their hands, or by any other means. "We who devote our time and our energy to working with persons with aphasia have long been aware that it is false to assume that conventional language constitutes the total range of our means of expression. The truth is, however, that to transcend this stage, one must first admit the obvious — that the person with aphasia should not just be considered someone who lost the use of speech, but rather as an individual with a distinct personality. The personality must be accepted the way it is, and must be used to the patient's advantage. This implies a respect and appreciation for both the individual's personality and his environment. The results obtained would otherwise be inconceivable if these conditions were not met."

THE WILL TO BE CURED

Through these observations and testimonies, it becomes clear that, notwithstanding the value of therapy, the patient's will to be cured is of prime importance. Guy Lorant[4], who co-wrote the book on Sabadel with Van Eeckhout, analyzed this issue, and referred to it as: "A vast topic." Two comments will be presented to complement what has been written above. First, there are evidently cases where even innovative approaches to the illness will not suffice to cure patients. These cases, however, are rarer than we would tend to believe. Secondly, patients must also make an effort. Consider the fact that, for a while, Sabadel shared a room with another person with hemiplegia. As soon as this man was faced with a problem he could not resolve, rather than exerting himself, he would snap his fingers to summon his wife for help.

The next step is to ask ourselves an even more basic question, one which we will not attempt to answer: What is the mysterious force that impels some people to survive, while others give up the ghost as soon as death beckons? Life instinct and death instinct, are they vying for supremacy at this very moment? Consider, for example, the case of Norman Cousins, the American who, despite a bleak prognosis, successfully recovered from his illness and later described his struggle in his inspirational book: *Anatomy of an Illness: Reflections on Regeneration.*

On the other end of the spectrum is the case of Fritz Zorn, the young Swiss author of a poignant account called *Mars.* The book describes how he allowed himself to be slowly devoured by cancer in an effort to escape a world in which he could never belong due to inadequate preparation. Since, fortunately perhaps, there is no definitive answer to the question of who survives, we prefer to imagine that Sabadel, during his illness, was driven by the urge to preserve an elusive quality found in each person that, as Malraux wrote, makes every person unique: *L'homme est l'homme, crée, invente et se conçoit.* (Man is man, he creates, invents and conceives himself).

These highly diverse perspectives are presented here to encourage the family and friends of the persons who suffer from aphasia-related linguistic and physical deficits to manifest more enthusiasm, willingness, and optimism. The alterations of body perception which complicate the patient's condition are not characteristic of all types of aphasia. In fact, as Luria[5] proposed:

> "Paroxysmic alterations of the body image (for example having the impression that one foot or hand has grown immensely, or that the shape of the head has changed) reflect damage to the systems in the parietal lobe. A precise analysis of this symptom reveals that pathology of the parietal-occipital region can induce visual and spatial disturbances which create a paroxysmic deformation of objects whose shapes and dimensions are perceived as being transformed (micro-, macro-, and metamorphopsia)."

Persons with aphasia are often overcome by feelings of degradation, regardless of their age at the onset of the illness. Whether viewed as a physiological, linguistic, or psychological problem, or as difficulty in social situations which may necessitate psychiatric intervention, to this day the motor deficits caused by aphasia are still considered a challenge to physical medicine and its related disciplines that have appeared in the past few decades to treat the diverse repercussions of severe strokes.

REFERENCES

1. Alajouanine, T.: *L'aphasie et le langage pathologique,* J.B. Baillière et fils, Paris, 1968.
2. Alajouanine, T.: Valéry Larbaud sous divers visages, Gallimard, Paris, 1973.
3. Froment, J.: Comment un aphasique incomplètement rééduqué donna dans l'aviation de combat, des preuves irrécusables de son intégrité psychique. *Journal de médecine de Lyon,* **mars,** 1942.
4. Lorant, G.: **in** *L'homme qui ne savait plus parler.* Sabadel. Nouvelles éditions Baudinière, Paris, 1980.
5. Luria, A.-R.: *Les fonctions corticales supérieures de l'homme,* P.U.F., Paris, 1978.
6. Sabadel: *L'homme qui ne savait plus parler.* Sabadel. Nouvelles éditions Baudinière, Paris, 1980.
7. Van Eeckhout, P.: **in** *L'homme qui ne savait plus parler.* Sabadel. Nouvelles éditions Baudinière, Paris, 1980.

CHAPTER 4

THE PSYCHOLOGICAL EFFECTS OF APHASIA

P.-Y. LÉTOURNEAU

THE IMPORTANCE OF COMMUNICATION

Humanity is presently in the post-industrial era, which some call the "communications age." In our society today, communications are omnipresent and indispensable. The many examples in our surroundings include the multitude of cable channels, interactive television, computers that can talk to each other, and telephones which have invaded every room in the house, the office, and even cars. Everything is moving at an accelerating pace, and distance is seen as less and less of a barrier to instantaneous communication. Communications have become the underlying force behind progress.

Under such conditions, it is easy to imagine the *stigma* that an individual can suffer when he or she can no longer communicate effectively. That person is immediately disconnected, limited, and disabled. To us, as speaking beings, language is more than just a practical tool; it is an integral part of our personal identities. It is well known that language conservation is an important issue for peoples such as French speakers in Quebec or certain European populations with the 1992 accord. Language often symbolizes group identity. Likewise, through communication individuals can profess their intelligence, alter their environment, and assert their existence. People who cannot speak are isolated from reality, and are deprived of a portion of their "humanity."

The term **"person with aphasia"** conveys the impression that it is the entire person that is affected or disabled by aphasia. That is, as if the whole person were impaired instead of just the capacity to read or to communicate. The objectives of this chapter are to explore, through clinical observations, the various psychological characteristics of the person with aphasia.

CLINICAL EXPERIENCE

For the past twenty years, we have been working with patients with aphasia, mostly stroke victims. We treated more male patients than female, and most were between the ages of 50 and 70. We have also worked with younger patients who acquired aphasia following a brain injury or tumor.

Our clinical experience to date has not been oriented towards the study of aphasia per se, but rather towards an understanding of the psychological experience of persons with aphasia; we aim to provide assistance for them, as well as for their families and friends.

In general, physical rehabilitation and speech therapy are considered the primary goals of treatment for persons with aphasia. Yet experienced therapists argue that the success of aphasia therapy largely depends on the patient's psychological state. For this reason we strive to be sensitive to the emotional and psychological responses of the patients in our care. Given the complexity of the psychological factors, it is sometimes tempting to neglect these problems, even if they persist after months of therapy, creating major obstacles for the persons with aphasia, their family, and friends. Furthermore, throughout rehabilitation, the patient's emotional problems can undermine the effectiveness of treatment.

It is with great modesty that we present the fruits of our labor to our colleagues in the aphasia treatment field. We also hope that our observations will promote a better understanding of the psychological effects of aphasia in specialists from various fields, family members, and perhaps even persons with aphasia themselves.

APHASIA: A DRAMATIC EXPERIENCE

Aphasia is probably the most serious disability of all the repercussions of brain injuries. Its symptoms — intellectual and emotional disturbances — can affect the patient on personal, social, and economic levels. In many cases, the treatment of aphasia is difficult and the results are uncertain, especially in elderly patients who cannot learn quickly and who are more likely to suffer relapses or deterioration of the illness. The same cannot be said for younger patients with aphasia, for whom the prognosis is generally rosier — that is at least what we would prefer to believe. For these young patients, the illness is perceived more dramatically. The attending staff must therefore keep in mind the importance and the necessity of developing a rehabilitation program that will take into account the various aspects of the person who has been affected by aphasia.

Most patients, especially stroke victims, are over age 50, i.e. in the second half of their lives, at the onset of aphasia. It is a golden age, a time when they enjoy greater freedom: they are often retired, their children have left the home, and they feel that the time has come to enjoy themselves!

Even though everyone knows that the *human machine* will slowly deteriorate with age, we all hope this process will occur very late in life. In the meantime, we feel young at heart and engage in activities such as physical fitness, sports, and travel. Aphasia hammers in the reality of aging in a single sudden blow. Patients seemingly age overnight. And they thought this only happens to other people! It is almost like dying.

Each stage of life poses difficulties and challenges which, once overcome, lead us to the next phase of our development. Usually, we are able to prepare ourselves for the next step, to see it coming. But who can be prepared for hemiplegia and aphasia?

What can persons with aphasia hope for when such a misfortune has arisen at this point in their lives? Why struggle, what do they have to gain, and what implications does this illness have for their future? Does life have something else to offer other than defeat and the further loss of integrity?

These persons and their family and friends have no alternative but to think that an injustice has occurred; this reaction is inevitably manifested by feelings of impotence, disbelief, frustration, and anger. There are so many unanswered questions. The occurrence of aphasia is one of the most distressing experiences in life. Some say that it borders on utter terror.

APHASIA AND THE PERSONALITY

Aphasia can bring about such drastic changes that people may wonder if the patient with aphasia is really the same person. The impact of the illness can be so severe that it becomes the predominant element in the patient's daily life as well as in therapy. Therefore, because these changes exact such a toll on the patient's quality of life and the prognosis for therapy, it is essential that these persons receive the attention they deserve.

These frequently observable changes in persons with aphasia can largely be accounted for by the individual's reaction to the illness (the emotional response to the realization of loss). The psychological reactions to aphasia may also be compounded, to varying degrees, by damage to the control and production mechanisms of the cognitive, perceptive, and emotional functions of the brain. Granted, it is sometimes difficult to determine whether the person's maladaptive behavior is a consequence of the emotional reaction to aphasia, or if it is directly linked to the brain damage itself.

In other words, the personality changes that can be observed in persons with aphasia have dual origins: Firstly, changes caused by the brain damage itself (for example, a frontal syndrome) and, secondly, those which stem from the patients' reactions (e.g. depression) as they confront their limitations. At this point we would like to stress the importance of the emotional reaction as the causal factor in personality changes in persons with aphasia.

The personality and behavioral alterations can be influenced by several variables or factors that can affect their intensity. Below, we will present a discussion of some of these variables.

Factors that May Influence Psychological Responses

In general, the psychological problems of persons with aphasia are influenced in particular by the severity and duration of the symptoms linked to aphasia and the concomitant physical disabilities. The individual's personality before the illness is also an important factor because a person with aphasia will tend to use the same coping mechanisms to deal with or adapt to the illness as the ones resorted to in the past.

Note that it is not uncommon to encounter persons with aphasia whose personalities change radically as a result of the illness. People who were formerly calm and rational may become anxious and labile, while others, good-natured, may turn aggressive, and so on. The changes may be so pronounced that the patient is barely recognizable.

In our opinion, it is the patients' *perceptions* of their limitations and the *significance* that these limitations acquire for them that will determine the specific nature of their emotional reactions, taking into account, of course, the circumstances at the time aphasia surfaces. Obviously, the patient must first *perceive* in order to *react.* This perception may not be present in cases of anosognosia or following severe injury.

In many cases, psychological responses may intensify as the persons with aphasia become more aware of the severity and the nature of their disabilities. Family members report: "Ever since he recovered physically, he seems to be more depressed." Here, although the subject seems to be recovering in general, the fact that he is simultaneously growing increasingly aware of his limitations can lead to discouragement. These feelings may coincide with the persons' return home, or when they confront their previous way of life.

The general situation of the person with aphasia, i.e. age, occupation, the presence or absence of a spouse or family members, the financial situation, and even social status all affect the way in which the person will react to aphasia and perceive his limitations.

The importance of language in the person's life can also be an influential factor. Actors, writers, and teachers have all expressed frustration and misery over not being able to use the tool which was previously so primordial in their lives.

The nature and the extent of the brain lesion responsible for aphasia also serve to explain the psychological reactions of persons with aphasia. The injury may alter other aspects of the patient's life by impairing motor functions, sensation, perception, memory, thinking processes, etc. These effects also tend to tarnish the patient's self-perception and dampen future aspirations. Other factors which account for variations in individual reactions to the illness include: The intellect and level of maturity of the patient, previous knowledge of aphasia, the sudden appearance of symptoms, the reactions of other people in the patient's environment, as well as personal values and religious beliefs. It is exceedingly rare to encounter individuals such as one of our former patients, who considered language to be essentially a capacity that had been lent to him, for which he was grateful to have had such extensive use over so many years!

Aside from the various elements mentioned above, we feel it is important to stress the predominant role of certain specific factors on the emotional condition of the person with aphasia. These include the prognosis, the quality of patient management by the family as well as the attending staff, and the quality of life that the persons can envision in their immediate future (for example, the question of returning home, continuing with favorite activities, etc.).

The Most Common Psychological Reactions

Kurt Goldstein, one of the founding fathers of neuropsychology, used the term "catastrophic reaction" to describe the psychological profile (or response to their condition) of persons with aphasia and hemiplegia. He believed that the reaction could be described as an acknowledgement of biological failure, rather than a depressive state induced by the patient's realization of his or her limitations.

As mentioned above, the emotional reactions associated with aphasia have two sources: One linked to the anatomic-physiological damage to the brain (neurological explanation), and the other arising from the persons' evaluation of their limitations in view of their general condition (psychological explanation). The paragraphs below will deal chiefly with the second type of reaction.

When individuals find themselves in new situations, or facing a loss or major uncertainty, they will generally respond as if they were exposed to a physical danger. Usually, patients will feel anxious or distressed. They will try to confront this new reality in order to recover their former equilibrium as quickly as possible. These emotions or worries indicate to the body that certain needs are not being sufficiently met. Most of the time, in persons with aphasia, such emotions are legitimate under the circumstances. It is in the way that these worries are experienced and the manner in which the strategies to regain equilibrium are utilized by the patient that the distinction between normal (useful) or abnormal (useless or even harmful) behavior can be made.

The psychological and behavioral responses listed below reflect the clinical profiles of patients during the first few months after the onset of aphasia (on average between six and twelve months). Note that the effectiveness of these attitudes or coping mechanisms is not necessarily evident; furthermore, some reactions serve as defense mechanisms to offset loss, failure, or the threat of an even greater misfortune to come.

Anxiety

Persons with aphasia often experience abnormally high degrees of anxiety (over fears of a relapse, death, or not being able to understand what is happening to them). They must confront the most traumatic situation in their lives, and their arsenal is limited. They also fear the unknown, an uncertain future, not being like before, and the loss of loved ones. They might also worry about losing their homes or not being able to return to work. It is impossible to imagine the upheaval that is taking place in such a person's life. The greater the awareness, the more the patient's anxiety increases until it can reach epic proportions. For this reason, prompt intervention is necessary to respond to the patient's urgent needs.

Denial

The reality of the condition of patients with aphasia is so traumatic that sometimes it is preferable for them to deny it, to be blind to it. Denial, or the refusal to recognize physical and psychological limitations, to pretend that nothing has happened, allows patients to gain time and to adapt gradually to reality. Denial can also protect patients from becoming depressed.

Note that this type of denial is psychological in origin and differs from anosognosia induced by posterior lesions, sometimes seen in persons with aphasia.

Caution is in order when confronting persons with aphasia with their denial behavior. Sometimes the surfacing of hope or unrealistic expectations can temporarily aid the rehabilitation process; it is at least preferable to severe depression. In the long run, however, denying one's limitations and entertaining unrealistic hopes can only have negative repercussions on treatment. How can one go about effectively treating someone who is convinced that he is in no need of help?

Regression

Apparently, in some cases, the person with aphasia will resort to less evolved or less sophisticated behavior patterns in an effort to adapt. Damage to the cognitive processes may also increase the possibility of regression in patients with aphasia who tend to exhibit psychological limitations. If we also consider other types of behavior resulting from lack of coordination or apraxia, it should come as no surprise that families often mistakenly assume that the person with aphasia is living a *second childhood.*

Egocentrism and Infantilism

When it comes to satisfying their needs, persons with aphasia doubtlessly place priority on basic needs such as eating, drinking, and sleeping which must be met on the spot (the patients require instant gratification). This is an ideal breeding ground for narcissism, especially when compounded by the persons' difficulty in visualizing situations globally. The family naturally concludes that the person is childlike. Naturally, even when they display inappropriate behavior, persons with aphasia still deserve our full respect as adults.

Damage to the Self Esteem

Persons with aphasia feel profoundly wounded. They may even lose their sense of identity. They may witness the disappearance of many of the activities which granted them importance or prestige, and their income and social status are significantly lowered. Their sources of self-confidence are temporarily blocked and some may never be reinstated. They may be unable to fill their former familial or social roles. The spouse or colleagues must fill **their shoes.** How can they be themselves, man or woman, or simply exist without being able to communicate adequately, without being able to share their inner turmoil, without working to their former capacity and possibly even without understanding what is going on around them?

Solitude and Isolation

Damage to self esteem and the difficulty communicating with others lead persons with aphasia to withdraw from social contact. The fear of rejection by family and friends can also drive them towards isolation. The patient's heightened sense of solitude can bring on feelings of sadness and depression, and simultaneously decrease opportunities to improve language skills and the adoption of alternative forms of communication.

Emotional Lability

Since the brain injury may lower inhibitions and reduce the ability to control emotions, it is not uncommon to observe persons with aphasia who tend to cry at inappropriate times. This behavior is not always associated with the appropriate emotional state. Perhaps the person is experiencing a rapid succession of emotions which are not motivated by actual circumstances. Other persons appear to be in a state of total indifference; they seem detached and even euphoric, as if they were impervious to harm, and as if they were living in the best possible world and looking through rose-colored glasses!

Aggression

Persons with aphasia are easily irritated due to their low tolerance of frustration. For these patients, the sources of frustration are abundant and, since they are often unable to control their emotions, it is not surprising that they sometimes become aggressive. For some people, aggression becomes a means of controlling their environment or asserting themselves. Inevitably, it is the people in close contact with the patient who become the victims; not because they deserve it, but only because they are present at the time of the aggressive outburst. It is preferable not to react to this show of aggression with anger or reciprocal aggression, because the person with aphasia will become considerably more disturbed. Usually if the person is distracted, this type of behavior will be curtailed. From our experience, we have found that asocial behavior patterns typified by aggression are more common among those who suffer head trauma than among stroke victims.

Shame and Guilt

The sense of being deprived of some of their human dignity may induce feelings of shame in patients with aphasia. The patients are often ashamed of what they have become and may feel utterly worthless. They might feel guilty about being a burden on family, friends, and colleagues because of their physical and psychological disabilities. If the family and friends do not fully understand the etiology of the person's deficits, they may also be ashamed of the person with aphasia, and be reluctant to be seen in public with him or her.

Dependence and Passivity

Given all that has happened to them, it is not surprising that persons with aphasia are tempted to resign themselves and entrust themselves to the care of others. The feeling of loss on many levels may induce, in these persons, a heightened need for affection and a search for secondary gains. Sometimes the limitations are such that, for a time, the person with aphasia has no choice but to depend on others. The patient may consider this a severe blow to the self esteem and may subsequently become aggressive or discouraged.

Lack of Inhibition

Due to either impaired judgement or a lack of control over emotional and sexual needs, people with aphasia may behave inappropriately, flouting social norms with their lack of both consideration and inhibition.

The 'All or Nothing' Principle

The psychological state of the person with aphasia is so precarious that the slightest success may be grounds for euphoria, while a failure may be magnified in importance, causing utter discouragement and removing all motivation to continue with the activity at hand. In some cases, refusal to engage in a given task or activity may be explained by the fear of failure. For this reason, it is important to propose less challenging activities at first to build the patient's confidence.

The manifestations and reactions described above may be observed to a greater or lesser extent, depending on the severity and duration of the symptoms, the reactions of loved ones, and the quality of support offered to the person with aphasia. Other factors include the promptness and the quality of the therapeutic approach used by the rehabilitation team, the prospects for the future and the residual capacities of the patient.

Anatomical and Clinical Correlations

Researchers have long strived to associate specific psychological behavior of patients with aphasia with the particular locus of the lesion. While it is essential to keep in mind the uniqueness of each case, it is nonetheless true that, as a rule, some psychological reactions tend to be more prevalent than others. This may depend on whether the injury is situated in the anterior or posterior regions of the dominant hemisphere.

In cases of anterior or prerolandic lesions, often associated with Broca's aphasia, it is common to observe patients whose language comprehension is relatively adequate, but whose verbal performance is quite disturbed.

As a result, these patients tend to shun activities that involve communication. They withdraw at the slightest provocation and communicate minimally and only to express basic needs. Persons with aphasia obviously experience a great deal of frustration, and although they may tend to anger easily, most often they appear helpless, powerless, and depressed. Kurt Goldstein used the term "catastrophic reaction" to describe these patients' reaction to their aphasia.

Lesions in the posterior or retrorolandic areas, often associated with Wernicke's aphasia, are known to induce language comprehension deficits. In many cases, patients are hardly aware of their disability, as if they did not realize that their comprehension is impaired. Moreover, it is not unheard of that they may appear indifferent to what is happening to them, or go so far as to deny any symptoms. Some of these patients experience euphoric or paranoid episodes.

Note that this type of categorization must be used with caution, and only as a guideline. Indeed, only attentive observation, valid assessment, and information on the patient's former personality can provide a realistic clinical picture of each person with aphasia that enters treatment.

The Grief Response

Grief is usually defined as pain or sadness that one experiences upon a death or a tragic event. By extension, the term "grief response" can be used to describe the stages in the psychological adaptation process that follow a loss.

Persons with aphasia can be said to be "grieving" for their lost functions. The loss, however, is by no means limited to mere speech or comprehension deficits. These persons also face the loss of self-esteem, familial and social roles, income, participation in cultural activities, sports and social events, and even their future aspirations.

The family, too, faces the loss of a dear member, or at least the person they knew and loved. The family must learn to love someone else, someone who, in many cases, is disabled. The grief response is a complex phenomenon which varies widely between individuals. For example, we know that people react differently when faced with the death of a loved one. The characteristics of the ensuing grief are contingent upon a number of factors such as the relationship with the deceased and the circumstances of death. Persons with aphasia also grieve as they come to grips with their losses. According to the significance that they attach to their loss, they pass through different stages before being able to adapt to their new condition. These steps towards adaptation may vary in length and intensity between individuals. The stages of the grief response can be summarized as follows:

- beginning of the awareness and initial shock;
- period of shock absorption, avoidance, or strong reactions;
- rationalization of symptoms, and first steps towards autonomy;
- adaptation, integration of limitations, and start of a new life.

The manifestations of the grief response are influenced by several variables. Here are the most common factors for patients with aphasia:

- the extent of the limitations and the disability;
- psychological implications of the loss of language;
- other losses associated with aphasia (for example, loss of prestige, income, and family or social roles);
- nature of the prognosis (level of autonomy), or projected length of time for recovery;
- level of maturity and resourcefulness;
- quality of care and support from family members and the attending staff;
- future plans or substitute activities, as compared with the patient's aspirations.

It is commonly believed that grief eventually subsides and disappears. This is generally true since, with time, people adapt to the loss and find other ways of meeting their needs. As well, the grief response tends to diminish in proportion to the improvements seen in the patient's overall physical condition.

Passing through the stages of grief is like solving an equation in terms that had previously been beyond one's grasp. Soon after the onset of aphasia, the only thought on the patient and the family's mind is "if only everything could be the way it was before." The notion of "like before" is omnipresent in rehabilitation. Most often, it represents the goal of treatment, the reason for expending all efforts and trying everything humanly possible. Suddenly, the lost abilities are all that matter, nothing else exists. The patient is seemingly inconsolable if those functions cannot be restored.

Rehabilitation experts are well aware of how difficult it is, during this period, to motivate patients to exert themselves to reach an objective that often falls short of "like before." In fact, it is only when the patients abandon the dream and realistically consider the possible that progress is truly attainable. At this stage, the tendency to deny the illness, to pretend as if nothing ever happened, can be seen as an attempt to resurrect the past, to avoid being confronted by an awareness that might be overwhelming, or too painful.

During this process, it is preferable to speak of *adaptation* to rather than *acceptance* of the loss. The latter word connotes resignation, defeat, and passivity, while *adaptation* is a more active term, and, in our opinion, conforms more closely with the inner experience of persons with aphasia. How can the unacceptable ever be accepted?

Depression

These days, the word depression is used to describe a panoply of psychological conditions. As soon as someone is not feeling cheerful, we say that he is *depressed*. In fact, in some cases, depression can be considered a normal reaction. It is only considered pathological when it is manifested in excessive proportions. One of my patients reported to me that he was depressed when he suffered from aphasia for a few months following an operation to remove a brain tumour. Who would not find such a loss traumatic?

For persons with aphasia, the depressive phase that often surfaces temporarily can be considered normal (adaptive) if it represents a psychological reaction due to the realization of a major loss. This transitory depression, brought on by any significant loss, is quite preferable to denial of the illness. Here, if the reaction is proportional to the loss, it should be considered as sadness or disappointment rather than as actual depression.

Patients can be diagnosed as depressed in cases where the outer loss, i.e. aphasia, arouses a profound sense of inner loss. This loss may be real or symbolic, and may exacerbate unresolved conflicts or other fears in the patient's mind such as the fear of death, rejection, being helpless and dependent like a young child, not being loved any more, not to love or appreciate oneself, or fear of abandonment and an uncertain future. The diagnostic term "depression" can thus be used in cases where the patient's symptoms and behavior are disproportionate with the extent of the deficits.

For example, in patients predisposed to depression (with a depressive nature), aphasia will heighten the feelings of loss and worthlessness, and may subsequently induce actual depression. In this case, the endogenous depression is triggered by a new setback.

Most often, depression is characterized by the following symptoms:

- generalized slowing (physical and psychological);
- generalized indifference and lack of energy;
- low self-image, sense of guilt;
- withdrawal from activity and social interaction;
- physical and emotional fatigue, apathy;
- difficulty in deriving pleasure from life;
- inability to be happy and to plan for the future; no enthusiasm;
- lack of motivation and a tendency to give up at the first sign of failure;
- high levels of anxiety, insomnia, loss of appetite, and sexual desire;
- 'teary eyes' on frequent occasions;
- suicidal thoughts.

Sadness, disappointment, or, in some cases, depression, are all aspects of an individual's reaction to a loss. For persons with aphasia, these losses are numerous and serious: they affect the person through and through.

How does an individual come to define his identity and personal worth? In psychology, each theory on personality development offers a different answer to this question. Practically speaking, however, in a society that prizes productivity, success, and satisfaction at all costs, the value of an individual is usually determined by the ability to satisfy one's needs. One must also be active, competent, efficient, independent, and capable of getting along with other people, as well as living up to their expectations.

People who are unable to meet one or another of these requirements in life, may find their self-image, self-worth, and even their identity being called into question. Persons with aphasia must make a tremendous effort to resolve these problems in life, concurrently regaining energy and a satisfying equilibrium.

To reach this equilibrium, persons with aphasia must first traverse many painful stages. The behavior which characterizes these transitions is often difficult for the family to comprehend (e.g. apathy, anger, aggression, and self-mutilation). During this period, how should the person with aphasia be viewed? The former standards or criteria are no longer valid. The person as well as the family and friends must develop new means of assessing the person's value or importance as an individual.

The spouse or family members will wonder if the person with aphasia is really the same **person**; since the former personality is often nowhere to be seen. Therefore, it is difficult to still feel the same affection for the person. Some spouses or family members, however, may feel bound by unconditional love, but are nonetheless confronted by a major diminishment of their level of satisfaction from the person with aphasia. Counselling is often required in these cases.

Normally, the depression-related forms of behavior will dissipate together with the organic causes and as the individuals adapt to their new lifestyle. This adaptation will necessitate significant changes, especially with respect to values. Often, in order to cope, people must totally revise their approach to life.

After three months of therapy, one patient claimed that everything had become considerably easier for him from the day that he had stopped insisting that his life be the way it was before. He transcended from *requirement to preference.*

> "I would have preferred to recover my former communicative skills, but if this is no longer possible, I will adapt to my new reality. I will live my life vacation *style*, and value life's pleasures over productivity at all costs! I finally realize the difference between *being* and *doing;* I never knew that the former could be so enjoyable, so satisfying, and so calming. I managed to build a new identity, perhaps even a better one than before. At least I stopped running! From now on, all I want is to try my best to do things for the better. I am learning to live without conditions, by enjoying life without rules or formulas for success."

What a lesson in life!

It is this ability to redefine oneself that enables some elderly people to adapt easily to retirement, unlike those whose values center entirely around the family or work. Those who successfully adapt discover other sources of satisfaction in life such as exploring their surroundings, developing new interests, choosing the activities that make the day more enjoyable, reorganizing their time, testing new avenues, discovering nature, appreciating music and attending performances, and cherishing the presence of a pet or a loved one.

In most cases, depression gradually fades away. However, it may reappear or be rekindled by a new perception of one's limitations or by a sudden collision with reality. For example, depression often occurs when the rehabilitation team terminates the treatment of a person with aphasia. Patients are confronted with failure, and the idea that their condition will never really improve. They may think "There is nothing left for me."

For the person with aphasia, the surest way to beat depression is to fight and to strive to ensure that the after-effects vanish as soon as possible. Patients must also struggle internally in order to redefine their identity as a person of full value, despite the communicative limitations.

APHASIA AND SEXUALITY

Aphasia may disturb human behavior on many levels, including that of sexual behavior. Sexual behavior includes any form of courtship, as well as actual erotic and sexual activities. Often, the person exhibits inappropriate sexual conduct such as bursts of hypersexuality, or major fluctuations in sexual drive. These disturbances primarily concern the person with aphasia, but can easily affect the spouse or other family members.

Who should be Consulted for these Problems?

Despite the openness that prevails in recent years regarding sexuality, the act of discussing one's limitations or sexual problems is still considered taboo. If the person with aphasia or the spouse decide to tackle this issue, who should they consult? Should it be the doctor, the physiotherapist, the nurse, the psychologist, or the speech pathologist? Which specialist can best meet their needs?

We would suggest that the person with aphasia discuss this problem with the professional with whom he has built up a solid trusting relationship and who will be able to understand him best, despite his communicative difficulties. Normally, this professional will be able to reply to the patient or his spouse's questions; if not, he or she can refer the patient to a specialist who is more qualified to provide informative answers. Most often, a urologist or gynecologist can assist with medical questions, and a psychologist or social worker can solve queries relating to psychological difficulties or problems with relationships. Some rehabilitation centers have a professional on their staff whose particular role is to answer such questions. The person may be a sexologist or someone with particular training in a subject in which people cannot become experts overnight.

Sexuality: A Barometer

Sexual activity consists in a delicate and fragile rapport between two people. Marriage counsellors can attest to the importance of communication in a sexual relationship. It is understandable that the sexual problems of a person with aphasia may stem from his difficulty to clearly communicate his worries and needs. He may also misunderstand his partner's explanations or refusals.

Persons with aphasia may also express their sexual needs inappropriately. Their sexual behavior may reflect difficulties in controlling their drive and making sound judgments, or may symbolize the obsessive need to prove that they can still satisfy sexually and perform as before. It is also possible that a patient may use sexual activity to obtain gratification, e.g. warmth and tenderness, that become even more precious during this traumatic period.

The spouse's inability to respond to the partner's sexual advances may signal a change in the relationship or a change in attitude towards the person with aphasia. Often, the spouse can no longer recognize, in the person with aphasia, the cherished and desirable partner. The spouse may also experience a grief response. The couple's pleasurable sexual activity will usually be resumed once both spouses have adapted to each other, often on new terms.

Usually, when couples are relating well, sexuality can thrive even when one of the partners has limitations. Here, aside from its important role in reproduction and the survival of the species, sexuality also serves as a means of expression, communication, and as a learning experience. It is also associated with reassurance, joy, humor, and tenderness.

The Most Common Worries Regarding Sexuality

For individuals who engaged regularly in sexual activity before the onset of aphasia, there should be little change in sexual drive during the illness, apart from cases where the patient is suffering from severe depression characterized by a significant decrease in libido. For persons with aphasia, the behavioral changes will be manifested in the means of communicating sexual desires (e.g. through inappropriate propositions).

The issues below are often the focus of concern for persons with aphasia who consult specialists regarding their sexuality:

The Physical Aspect *(Medical or Genital Problems)*

Aphasia is rarely an isolated symptom. The person with aphasia often suffers from additional physiological symptoms related to his condition. The most common complaints regarding sexuality are: difficulty in achieving or maintaining erections, loss of sensitivity, inadequate vaginal lubrication, interruption of the menstrual cycle, compulsive masturbation, difficulty with sexual positions, difficulty reaching orgasm, the presence of spasms and contractions, and loss of sphincter control.

The Psychological Aspect

Aside from the physical aspects of sexuality, the associated emotions are also significant. The art of attracting, seducing, or convincing one's partner to engage in sexual activity is not always easy, even for able-bodied individuals. The person with aphasia is definitely at a disadvantage in this respect. The most frequently reported difficulties and worries include: finding and keeping a partner, anxiety and a constant need to affirm one's sexual capacities (persistent demands on the partner); feelings of rejection and low self-esteem if the spouse loses interest or refuses; lack of inhibition (inconsideration, and disrespect for societal norms on sexuality), and inappropriate propositions (wrong choice of a partner, wrong time, or unconventional form of request).

Personal Considerations

In principle, everyone, regardless of age, is entitled to engage in sexual activity that involves both partners in the giving and receiving of pleasure along with the release of sexual tensions.

Naturally, this activity can be enjoyed on many levels and to various degrees (passion versus tenderness and intimacy). Rather than be curtailed, sexuality should be adapted to the person's individual needs. Sexual activity may vary widely according to the person's age, previous experience, medical condition, and legal status.

It is obvious that a young man who suffered from a ruptured aneurysm during the sexual act will require special consideration from the health-care professional to guide him, as well as his partner, towards a return to an active sex life.

The Benefits of a Renewed Sex Life

If it is difficult to discuss sexual issues under normal circumstances, the situation becomes more complicated when one of the partners has aphasia. Specialists and the partner of the person with aphasia should keep in mind that it takes time and patience! Persons with aphasia are indeed capable of enjoying satisfying sexual activity, even if they must now use other forms of expression. Patients should not to be afraid to explore new possibilities once their physical condition has stabilized. They should be encouraged to be inventive in their sexuality and to stress satisfaction over performance. Their preferences may be subsequently redefined in terms of their capacities.

The benefits that a person with aphasia can derive from a satisfying sex life should not be underestimated. Sexuality is an alternative means of communicating certain emotions; it often alleviates depression, and boosts self-esteem as well. Many therapists will confirm that an improved sex life is directly linked to increased motivation in rehabilitation.

The Spouse

In occurrences of aphasia, it is not an exaggeration to state that the spouse and loved ones are also *victims*, since in many ways they are also affected by the illness. This is particularly true regarding sexuality. Sometimes the partner is as much in need of help as the person with aphasia. The spouse often faces many difficulties: How to resist the person's continual advances, how to adjust to the personality changes, how to cope with the inability to engage in sexual activity with the person with aphasia, how to remain faithful? What does the future hold? Should the spouse seek a divorce, start a new life? How should spouses handle their feelings of guilt and uncertainty? These are just a few of the questions that distress the spouses of persons with aphasia, at least during the first few months that follow the onset of the illness. Spouses must also adapt to substantial changes and make major decisions about the future, in particular the future of the relationship.

The influence of aphasia on the survival of the couple depends largely on the quality of the relationship between the spouses prior to the onset of the illness. In a successful marriage, the couple will most often confront the problem of aphasia with courage and determination, especially if the affected partner receives adequate professional support. In other cases, aphasia may be the final blow to relationships already fraught by serious problems, making the separation even more dramatic for the couple.

To conclude this discussion of sexuality and persons with aphasia, we must stress the importance of providing the couple with information, counselling with a qualified specialist, as well as the promise of rehabilitation. These elements will usually ensure positive results in this crucial sector of human activity.

APHASIA AND THE HELPING RELATIONSHIP

The therapeutic approach that we have developed for persons with aphasia is practically identical to the one used for other clients. It is important, however, for therapists to understand the persons' experience and adapt to their performance and comprehension deficits.

Our therapeutic approach features two levels, one intellectual, i.e. providing information, explaining the nature of the cognitive deficits, and the other emotional, which aims at empathic understanding. As in all forms of therapy, we believe that it is essential to establish and maintain a high caliber relationship with the person with aphasia. It is only once this relationship has been established that specific positive results can be anticipated. In the helping relationship with a person with aphasia, the quality of the relationship itself is often more significant than the objective help the therapist can offer.

The therapeutic relationship provides a climate where the person with aphasia can satisfy some of his basic needs (security, confidence, understanding, acceptance, and appreciation). In some cases, this is the only relationship which can offer non-judgmental respect and reassurance. The atmosphere is often sufficient to bolster their self-esteem and motivate them to minimize their limitations and exercise their residual skills. The inner resources of persons with aphasia, i.e. the urge to recover and to fight for survival can thus be harnessed. The person will ultimately declare: "I am worthy of progress."

Even though psychotherapy is verbal by nature, experienced therapists have been able to adapt their techniques to the limitations of persons with aphasia through the use of touch, monologues, role-playing, computers, writing, drawing, painting, and nonverbal tests which allow persons with aphasia to prove to those around them that they are not "crazy."

We believe that the helping relationship stimulates progress in the treatment of aphasia by reducing the length and intensity of the patient's psychological reactions. Emerging from a depression always heralds a major existential change of direction. If we consider that persons with aphasia must cope with limitations resulting from their brain injury, it is unrealistic to expect them to succeed unaided.

The therapeutic approach is based on a global view of the person, and can be integrated with other treatment methods. Furthermore, it provides other health-care professionals with information as to the patient's psychological condition. This approach involves the spouse and the family in addition to the patient with aphasia.

CONCLUSION

Aphasia is an upheaval that profoundly affects the whole person. Its severity should not be underestimated. The psychological problems stem from the privileged role of language in our society and the key role language plays in the definition of the personality and human identity.

To acquire aphasia is to suddenly lose both an important part of oneself and one's attachment to reality with no readily available means of compensation. While several specialists focus their treatment on the lost or impaired functions, it should be noted that others concentrate on the person with aphasia as a human being who is suffering and disoriented because of all that is happening.

To our knowledge, the most effective therapeutic strategies are those with client-centered approaches which take into account the psychological symptoms which inevitably accompany aphasia and which develop and apply techniques to reduce the limitations brought on by the symptoms of aphasia. To neglect one or another of these aspects will considerably (and unjustifiably) reduce the possibility of progress in the treatment of persons with aphasia as well as their families.

CHAPTER 5

APHASIA AND ARTISTIC CREATION

P. VAN EECKHOUT

INTRODUCTION

The problem of stimulating the creativity of a person with aphasia is not limited to the formulation of the therapeutic approach; therapists also must contend with factors relating to behavior and attitude.

As a person with aphasia becomes aware of his physical condition and his language impairment, he may overdramatize the situation, and drown himself in re-education. He abandons himself to the *total care* of the medical team, the family, and society. These institutions, though indispensable, ultimately deprive the person of his identity.

First the patient loses his dignity. Without dignity, there is no freedom. Without freedom, there is no responsibility, and without freedom, he is not accountable to anyone for his actions, including himself. He does not even have to take responsibility for his condition. Endure it? Hardly! He only has to be what he is: a person with aphasia.

These introductory statements may seem outrageous. Yet they will seem less so after you have read this chapter dedicated to artists or other artistically inclined persons with aphasia. The discourse that follows does not aim to spark creativity in persons with aphasia, but, rather, to revive the persons' former personality and, possibly to stimulate the creative process. This urge to awaken the artist within is inspired by the observations below.

CLAUDE B., ILLUSTRATOR

Tragedy

Claude B. is seated in a treatment room, opposite his speech pathologist. He is trying, or so it seems, to link two words in a sentence, an exercise known as sentence production. For example, the patient may be given the words "woman...sun." The speech pathologist is uneasy, embarrassed, somewhat pitiful, and seems to be in the grips of his worst nightmare.

A conversation in the corridor leading to the various offices reaches the therapist, who, overcome, attempts to drown out the merciless verdict with his voice. He repeats dumbly, like a broken record "What does the woman do in the sun?" Claude B., while repeating just as automatically, "My wife, my wife, . . . I . . . my wife," is nonetheless well aware that the conversation in the corridor concerns him and his aphasic condition. Unconsciously, he realizes that from now on, society has officially given him another identity, that of a person in his forties with aphasia. He also senses that in order to survive, he must relinquish his former identity; he must grieve for the man he used to be.

The actual conversation took place between Claude's wife and the psychologist, who was drawing conclusions based on the results of the neuropsychological examination of the patient after three months of rehabilitation. In short, the patient:

- spoke only upon request, with informative but reduced and agrammatical utterances (e.g. "hand bad")
- could not name adequately (two correct answers out of ten);
- could read only simple words;
- wrote with a scrawl, taking dictation with his awkward left hand;
- had severe comprehension problems (four mistakes out of ten in a pointing task);
- utterly failed the Binois-Pichot (synonym selection) test;
- displayed average performance in the Raven Progressive Matrices, and the REY figure was reproduced in the analytical mode.

The psychologist proposes that a complete reorganization is necessary. A training method must be found that would recuperate the patient's former abilities. He suggests that COTOREP[1] be contacted. The verdict strikes like a bullet: "I don't believe that he will draw again." To which Claude's wife spontaneously cries out "If he can no longer draw, he'll blow his brains out."

The speech pathologist is deeply disheartened by this exchange, which reaffirms his own assessment of Claude B.'s linguistic abilities. He had observed the following: no spontaneous language, and passive resignation interspersed with catastrophic reactions during rehabilitation exercises, all compounded by severe motor deficits.

The first act of this drama concludes with Claude B. in despair, and the speech pathologist crushed by his own failure.

Starting Over

With an authoritative, i.e angry tone, the speech pathologist asks Claude B. to draw his native village with his left hand. He wants Claude to perform immediately. In three minutes, the village "Sabadel," near Cahors, appears on paper (Figure 5–1.) This drawing symbolizes the reawakening of a personality. At this point, Claude B. has shed his identity as a person with aphasia for good, and has regained his true identity: A fortyish illustrator, cartoonist, and artist.

It is an imposing responsibility for language pathologists to face the task before them: The transformation of a mental vision into reality. Therapists must find it excruciatingly difficult to admit that they are often the jailer in the client's prison. The person with aphasia is confined to structured rehabilitation therapy, with bars built of lexical inventory and syntax. The result is an ultimate deprivation of

---

[1]French organization that assists disabled persons.

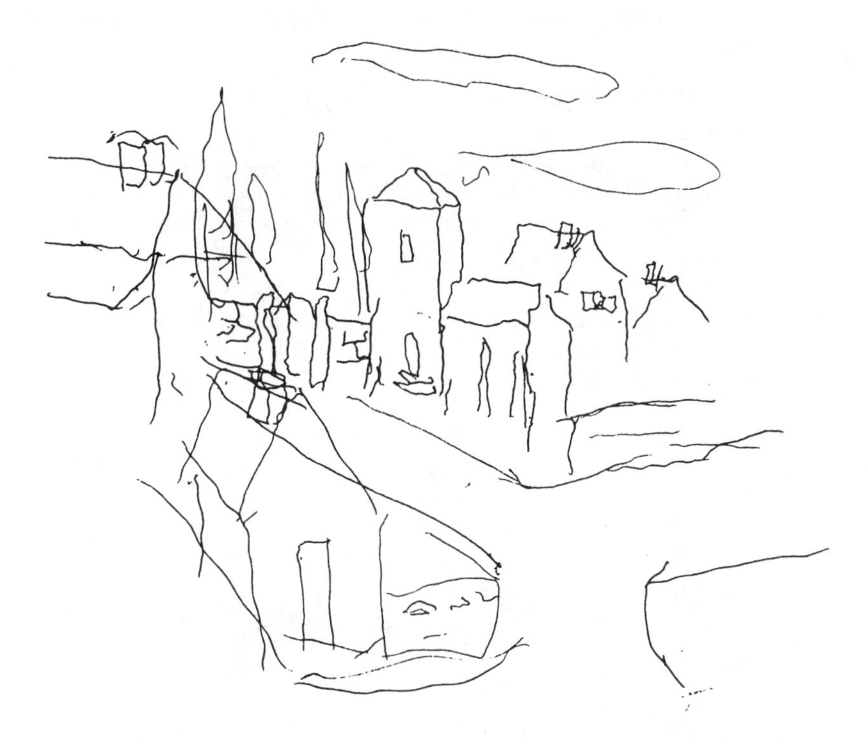

Figure 5–1

the person's freedom — the freedom to think of other things besides his disability.

Sabadel marked the start of a long journey, rich in experience, in questions, in changes of attitude, and power struggles. Claude B. also learned what it is like not to be respected for who one is, deprived of one's potential for creativity that can and must continue to thrive.

Drawing was subsequently proposed as a means of expression. This new start consisted of three stages:

Representational Drawing

Three months after the stroke, due to the severity of C.B.'s comprehension deficits and the need to utilize and educate the left hand, drawings are limited to the representation of various objects (Figure 5–2).

The Illustrated Account

C.B. is asked to illustrate a story which is narrated verbally (Figure 5–3). The story is well understood and humorously depicted. The cap-

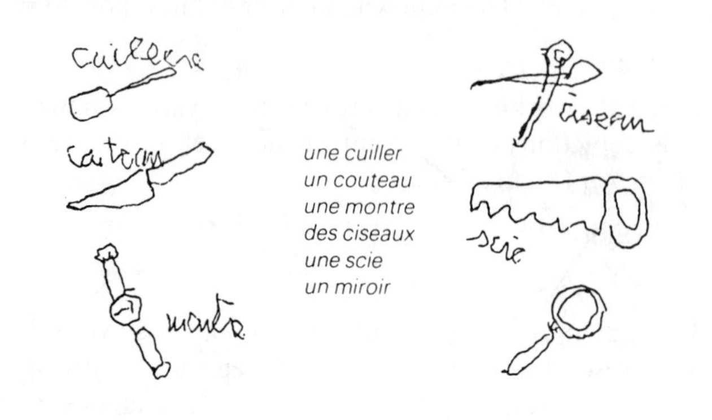

Figure 5–2

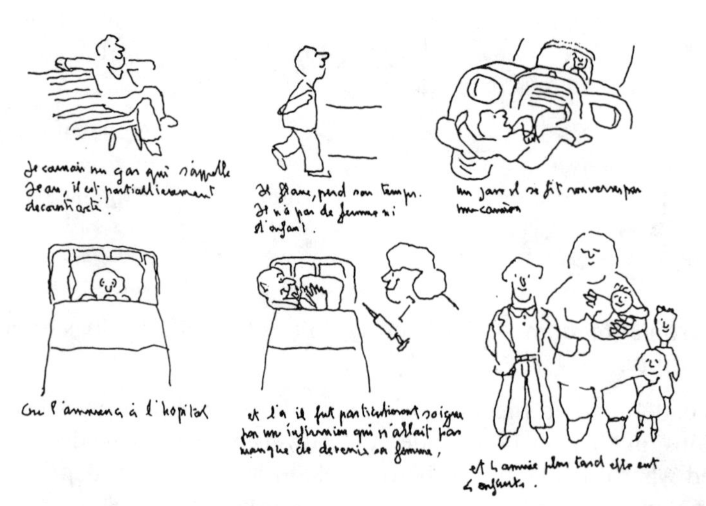

Figure 5–3

tions are not only explanatory, they also contribute to and complement the drawings.

Drawing: Self Expression

C.B. begins to recover verbal and graphic autonomy. He does not discuss his graphic expression, and is still dependent on the therapist. He does not voluntarily engage in personal creation. After having produced several illustrations of his family life, C.B. is asked to provide an illustrated account of his experiences from the onset of the illness

(Figures 5–4, 5–5, and 5–6). The result was a book entitled *L'homme qui ne savait plus parler*[1] (The man who no longer knew how to speak).

The Artist in 1989

C.B. is currently working as an illustrator for various newspapers. Of note are his depictions of the event of the week in the newspaper *Témoignage Chrétien* (Figure 5–7).

JEAN L., ORGANIST

Drama

J.L., right-handed, has been blind since the age of two, following glaucoma complicated by an eye infection. At age 10, he attended the boarding school l'Institution nationale des jeunes aveugles de Paris (the national institute for young blind people in Paris), and in two years learned to read and write Braille. Three years later, he mastered musical notation in Braille. At age 16, he devoted himself entirely to the organ and won first prize at the Conservatoire in 1930. By 1932, he was named master organist of a prestigious Parisian church organ. He later made numerous recordings. In 1983 he stopped composing, but continued to perform and to give lessons.

On July 1, 1984, he suffered a stroke[2]. During the execution of mass, he experienced a brutal suspension of verbal expression, accompanied by a lack of coordination in his right arm. The diagnosis revealed an infarct in the left middle cerebral artery. After 15 days in the hospital, the patient returned home. Oral expression was once again possible, but remained limited. The resulting comprehension deficits impaired communication and the patient could no longer read or write Braille. His musical abilities were affected for nearly a month.

By September 14 of that year, ten weeks after the stroke, the patient was receiving speech therapy at home. For two months, he was asked to play the organ at regular intervals. All of his musical abilities were subsequently noted. There were no observable motor and sensitivity impairments. A CAT-scan showed a broad hypodensity in the left temporal lobe, in particular Wernicke's region, as well as in the inferior region of the left parietal lobe.

Oral expression was disturbed in all modalities. Spontaneous expression was fluent, with no articulatory deficits. Intonation was also preserved. The patient had difficulty connecting syllables, leading to blockages and *"conduites d'approche"* (hesitations) and, less frequently, phonemic paraphasias (neologisms). Grammatical construction was varied, but nouns were rare, often replaced by circumlocutions or statements of failure. His speech, deficient in information, was considered jargon. For example, in response to the question "Do you like

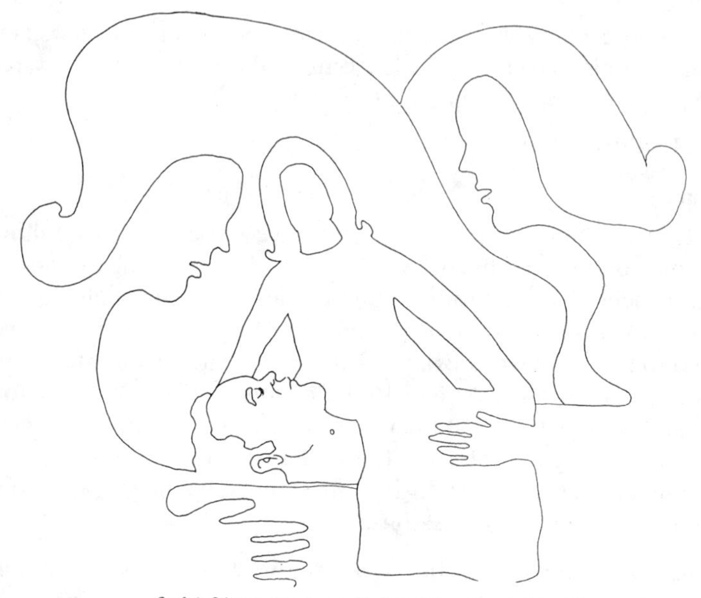
Ça fait 8 jours que je suis là, à moitié endormi, à moitié conscient...

Figure 5–4

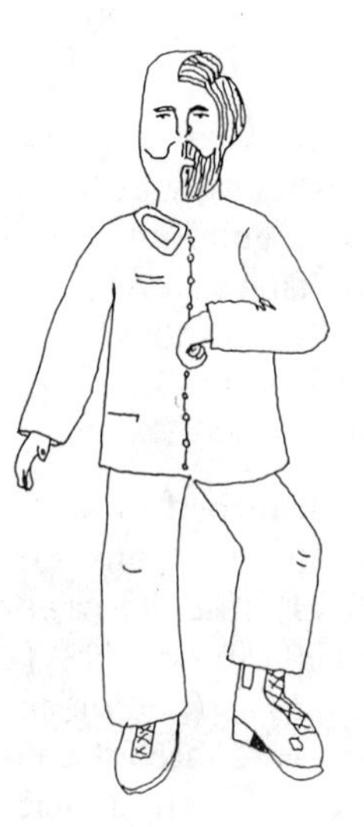

Figure 5–5

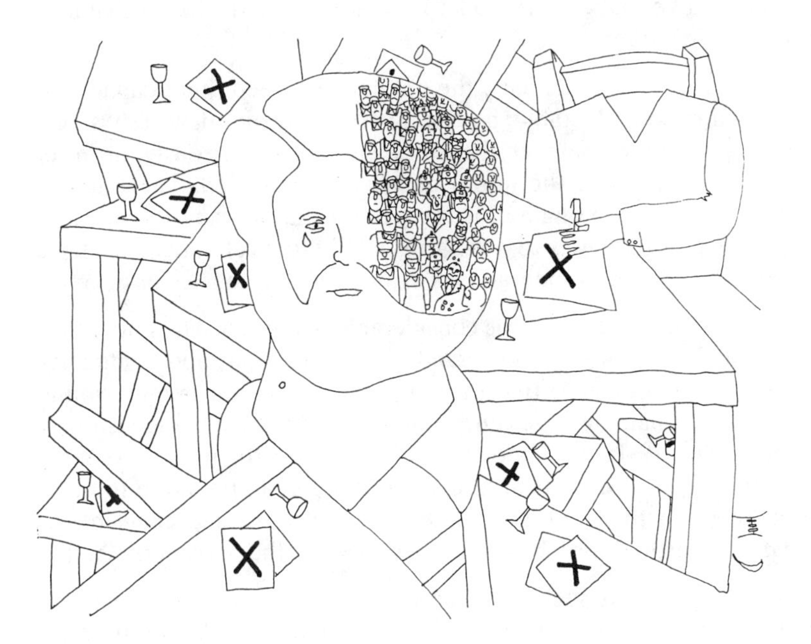

Figure 5–6

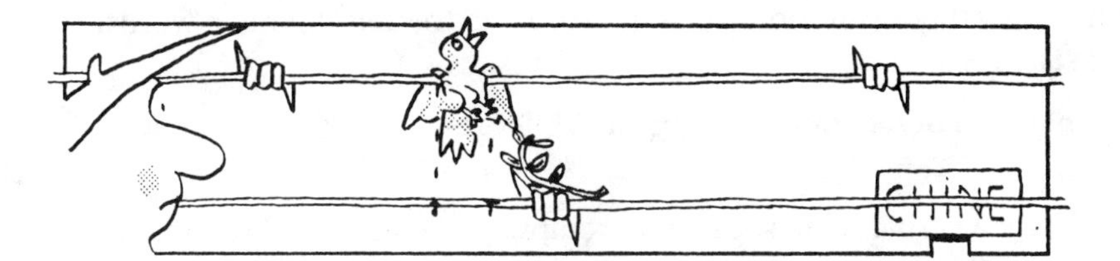

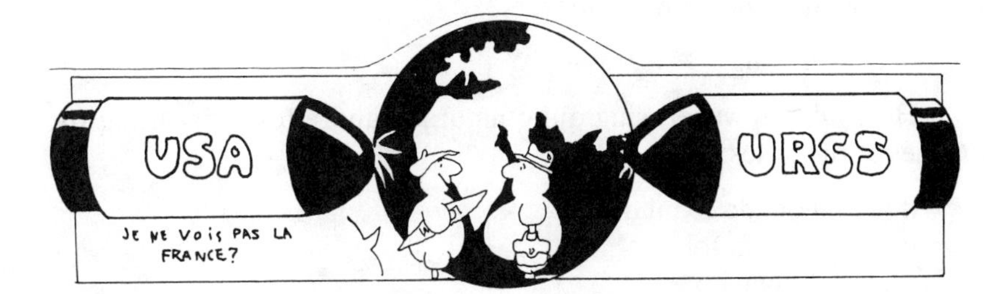

Figure 5–7

cheese?" the patient replied: "As for the machine of which when I drink things like that . . . Ah! O.k., I don't have what I like, I like best what is very good for me."

Despite his verbal deficits, the patient remained quite capable of humming a melody. Notably, he could very easily and flawlessly sing a song along with the names of the notes, either spontaneously, or in response to a request, if the initial notes were provided. These notes, however, could not be named if the patient did not sing them. Likewise, the use of the lyrics to a song revealed identical deficits to those described in relation to spontaneous expression, but to a lesser degree.

Verbal comprehension was considerably disturbed. The patient retained only the ability to understand simple questions and commands relating to everyday activities, thus allowing for basic communication. The individual naming of seven commonly used objects was also performed flawlessly. It was impossible, however, for the patient to name two of the previous objects at a time. Orders given in relation to these objects (e.g. put the comb on the key) were also incomprehensible to the patient. Furthermore, he was unable to name the parts of the body.

Verbal questions such as: "Can rain penetrate a good raincoat?" could not be answered. Yet the patient was quite capable of differentiating between similar words (good, wood) or homonyms, as well as non-words (cofa-cafo). Familiar noises and the voices of loved ones could also be identified. The patient experienced considerable difficulty repeating even monosyllabic words, extremely familiar words, and simple sentences.

Examination of the Patient's Musical Abilities

Singing

Upon a verbal request or with prompting, the musician was able to hum, mouth closed, any tune that he knew. He could not, however, provide the words, even when he knew them well. For example, the song *Frère Jacques:*

ma sa mère mer la mè la mère

"I can't say it. No."

He could, however, sing quite naturally and effortlessly using the names of the notes:

do re mi do, do re mi do
mi fa sol, mi fa sol,
sol la sol fa mi do
sol la sol fa mi do
do sol do, do sol do

When notes were played on the organ, he was able to name five or six while singing. He could also sing a melody after it had been played.

Identification

Jean L. was able to identify a number of musical pieces played by one of his students. Naturally, he had difficulty supplying the lyrics. Most often, he would sit at the organ to play a piece. His performances were flawless. For example, when a student played *La Prière* (The Prayer) by Franck, J. L. would exclaim "Yes, I know, it's the great, the great who says to God, to God, I pray, pray, pray, tray.."

Performance

He could perform pieces upon demand, reproduce short melodies directly on the organ, duplicate chords, and change octaves. He was also able to discern and correct false chords played by a student. The patient's sight-reading skills were also examined. Like all blind musicians, J. L. read with his left hand and played with his right. The various passages suggested were read and performed without difficulty.

Reading Music, Reading Words

J. L.'s case provides a fascinating and unique opportunity to study the relationship between reading musical notation and reading the alphabet and words. Braille is an ideal system for this purpose, since it uses identical configurations of dots to represent either letters or notes (Figures 5–8a and 5–8b). The patient could read neither words nor syllables, and was mistaken three out of four times in the identification of letters. In contrast, he was able to sing musical passages perfectly well by reading the notes. As soon as the patient was told that he was reading words, the same signs gave rise to failure or paraphasias. For example,

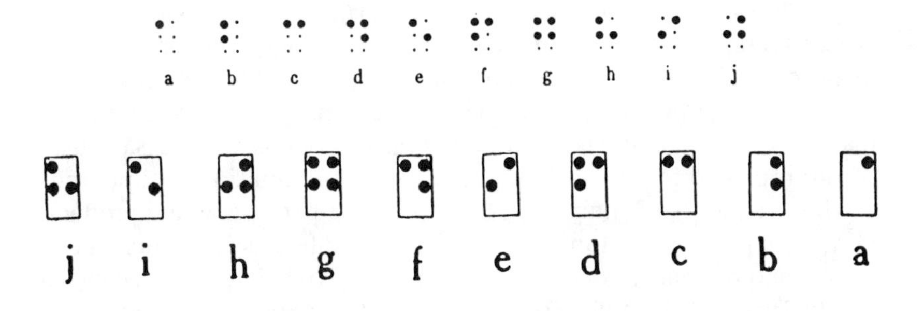

—The Braille alphabet read (upper line) and written (lower line), showing how the pattern of dots is reversed.

Figure 5–8a

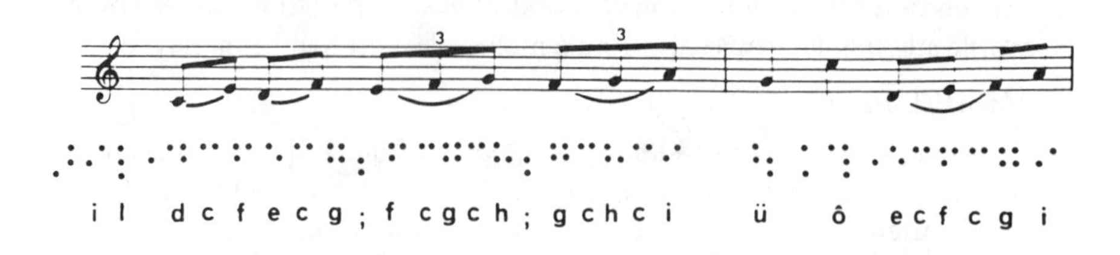

Example of a musical passage in Braille. The transcription of the signs into letters produces an unintelligible text.

Figure 5–8b

the notes "mi la re mi" were read. The corresponding word is "fief" which the patient read as: "pa fil."

The patient was perfectly capable of reading, without singing, the various notes of a musical passage. However, when faced with a written text, he was unable to connect letters and words. This dissociation was also found in repetition.

When asked to repeat homophone versions of notes "l'ami Rémi," he mistakenly replied "labi tavi." J. L. could transcribe musical notation of short melodies into Braille, but the transcription of short linguistic phrases resulted in abundant paragraphias.

The different modalities of information processing of the same system (Braille), depending on whether notes or phonemes were represented, constitutes a most striking example in favor of the argument that language and music are governed by independent functions in the brain.

J.L.'s adequate non-verbal, i.e. musical, performance allowed him to regain self-confidence, to play again, and to compose. He has written 32 compositions since his stroke (Figure 5–9). The "shattered" language function, which he considers a disability, is being dealt with in other ways. He aspires to improve his verbal performance. Along with his speech therapist, he selects therapeutic strategies. He occasionally comments critically on an exercise. For two years, he worked on self-correction. The use of prosody, the melody inherent in language, is the primal feature of this therapy. The underlying principle of this method is the use of the prosodic features of language (accentuation, intonation, and rhythm) as means of stimulating two processes: perception and production. The prosodic structure of utterances is modified; accentuation, intonation, and rhythm are deliberately simplified. Articulatory and acoustic features are exaggerated to offer the patient a simple and well-defined prosodic model, in which the individual elements are clearly differentiated.

Today, J.L. still uses circumlocutions to compensate for his word-finding difficulties. Yet he has virtually no difficulty communicating.

He discusses his problems with humor, and insists that his creativity is constantly being enriched.

MICHEL P., DEVOTED SINGER

Michel P. earns his living raising sheep. He is a noted singer, poet and, locally, a true artist, satirist, and anarchist.

In late 1983, he was found under his tractor which had been overturned in a car accident. For three months he was comatose. The brain scan revealed a lesion in the left Sylvian region. M. P. suffered from massive right hemiplegia and mixed aphasia with motor predominance. In his bed in the intensive care unit, M. P. would listen with earphones to his own compositions, and would tap the rhythm with his left hand on the metal bars of the bed.

For two years, he was rehabilitated, largely through music therapy, by a speech therapist in Limoges. The technique made almost exclusive use of intonation, rhythm, accentuation, and visual representations.

In December 1985, Michel P. arrived in Paris. His oral and written expression was intelligible, sometimes well structured, yet slow with articulatory difficulties. Verbal fluency was normal. Oral comprehension was satisfactory. He had come to Paris to learn to sing again — his main goal. M.P.'s personality made it impossible to turn down his requests, even though the task was daunting. He was asked to compose texts on aphasia and then to

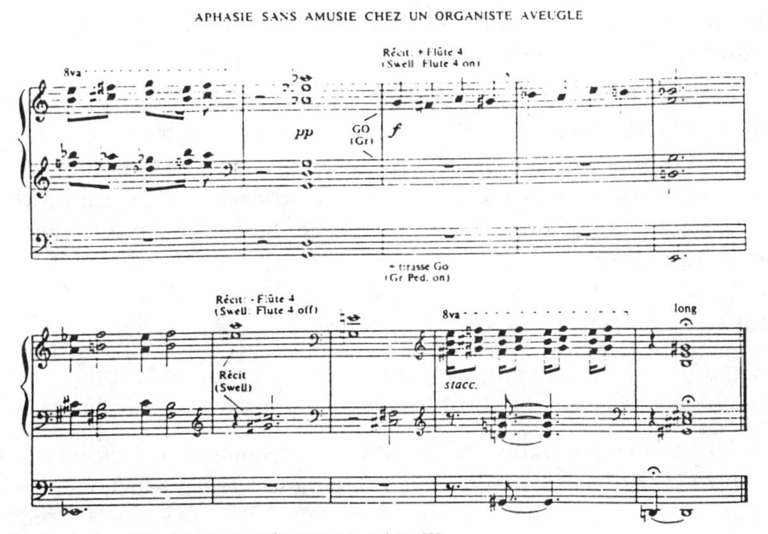

FIG. 8. – Extrait d'une pièce pour orgue composée par M. J.L. en juin 1985.
Extract of a musical piece for organ composed by M. J.L. in june 1985.

Figure 5–9

put them to music. He was also asked to sit in front of his window on the seventh floor, and to meditate on what he wanted to sing and on the many texts that would he have to write. Below is one of his many outlines:

"Looking out my window, my hopes are soaring higher, on the open road ahead, there's everything I desire."

With the help of the speech pathologist, he composed songs about aphasia, in order to reach a motivated audience that could be spurred into action. M.P. set his words to music with a guitarist from his old rock group. Thus highly technical articulation and vocal exercises efficiently had their effect, but over a long period of time. One of the speech pathologists responsible for this case, an individual who was highly committed to the project, provided therapy in the patient's home, while another professional worked with M.P. in the hospital. In 1986, *La Fondation de France* financed the production of a cassette. M.P. himself promoted this recording by visiting local radio stations and speech therapy conventions. Encouraged by his success, (M.P. sold 1000 cassettes on his own), he reformed a rock band in the summer of 1988 and recorded a selection of his old and new compositions.

In 1989, he gave up singing, considering that he met the challenge. He then began training as a sound engineer. He still enjoys writing, especially poems that describe the Love of Life. Here is an excerpt: "*Je sens qu'une vie faite de poèmes et de lumière s'échappe des sombres journées sans vie, qu'il faut à la nature donner de son soi et la laisser pensive, attendant avec impatience qu'elle hoche la tête pour dire qu'elle a compris.*"[2]

Michel P. is not alienated by his linguistic and physical disabilities. He knocks on doors, even on our own office door, to seek help, or more precisely, to ask us to listen, to recognize the satirist and the poet. Since then, that is since the outside world can look beyond M.P.'s hemiplegia and the slowness of his speech, he is striving for new successes, to surpass himself even further.

JEAN R., MUSIC LOVER

At age 76, Judge R., a music lover from early childhood, suffered from two consecutive infarcts which affected both cerebral hemispheres.

During hospitalization the patient was diagnosed as suffering from a loss of sensitivity in his right hand — a motor deficit which hampered

[2] "A life of poems and light banishes days somber and dead, give of yourself to Nature, let her meditate, then eagerly await; she understands, and nods her head."

grasping movements, a partially regressive Wernicke's aphasia, as well as severe paralytic dysarthria which required regular speech therapy.

After three months of re-education, his speech had returned to a normal level of complexity. The word-finding difficulty had practically disappeared. It was only the dysarthria that continued to impair the intelligibility of spontaneous expression. Mr. R. quickly regained his autonomy. His speech therapy essentially centered around the account of his imprisonment during the last war, as well as discussions of music. He heartily conversed on classical music, as well as on his own compositions, written in the POW (Prisoner of War) camps. He attempted to play the piano in order to recover agility in his fingers. He read *Le Monde* every day, and would listen to *France-Musique* or to records in the afternoon. In June 1989, Mr. R. began to experience urinary incontinence and ideomotor apraxia.

At 1 P.M. one Saturday, the speech pathologist visited Mr. R. in his new residence: a nursing home. He found him seated in an armchair, firmly bound by a sheet tied from behind. His face lit up when he saw the therapist and he immediately imitated with his left hand a pair of cutting scissors (the index and middle fingers spread and then closed, with the other fingers bent). He was signalling an immediate need: to be untied from the armchair. The speech therapist asked the nurse on call if he could bring the patient to the visiting area. The nurse then offered several words of caution: "The patient might do silly things; he was found in pyjamas at a bus stop; he wants to go home; he forgets himself..." Armed with this valuable information, the speech pathologist managed to accompany J.R. to the famous waiting room. He then gives him *Le Canard Enchainé*[3]. J.R. thanked him but, quickly enough, expressed a desire to listen to music. The therapist mentions Chopin and Liszt, and J.R. drums the fingers of his left hand as if playing notes on a keyboard.

Classical music is very meaningful to this patient. It had been a faithful ally during the most trying periods of his life. Because of actual or remembered classical music, the patient was able to experience intense feelings of freedom. Music was thus the privileged symbol of liberty. Without this artistic fervor, Mr. R. would not have had the energy to demand or to aspire towards autonomy.

How can one not despair when faced with this culturally and psychologically destitute environment, a setting where the last few years of life are empty of meaning? Hope can be seen in Mr. R.'s ardent music appreciation, which is the gateway for his deep desires and dreams of liberty.

---

[3] A satirical newspaper.

CONCLUSION

The first three examples illustrate the power of creativity in patients whose lives were previously devoted to art. They also reveal the effectiveness of creative energy to stimulate all of the person's capabilities. Creativity can also facilitate the restoration of language to levels comparable to the patient's former abilities.

The final example is a unique case. Mr. R. did not earn his living through art, it was not his profession. Music, however, is his passion. Four years in a POW camp in Germany were endurable thanks to music. Half a century later, he finds himself in a situation which he considered identical to his war-time experiences, and music naturally symbolizes freedom once again. Listening to Liszt and Chopin allows him to escape, the way it did in his previous experience. In this case, the patient's memory is creative and should be considered as such. As an artist remembers, poetry emerges. This is known as poetic analogy. The power of the imagination transcends the therapeutic method. J. R. imagines himself to be free, and in fact he is. He is no longer constrained by therapy.

The four examples above all involve the imagination. It is this **imagination** that the therapist must strive to stimulate. For example, it is not by merely asking the patient to name a bottle that the artist will be awakened. The inability to say a word creates an intellectual conflict. The artist is not governed by logic, but rather by emotion. Therefore, a distinct approach must be used. The rehabilitation of artists with aphasia requires in-depth research on their personality, and on personality in general. The family, especially the spouse — as the privileged partner — can provide information on the artist's past. Here, therapists must be exceptionally inquisitive, attentive to the slightest flicker of special interest in a particular area, and sensitive to creativity. They must understand that the identity, and thus the real life, of their patients is not confined to the ability to name words; in the case of artists in particular, it is defined on another level—that of the imagination.

REFERENCES

1. Sabadel: *L'homme qui ne savait plus parler.* Sabadel. Nouvelles éditions Baudinière, Paris, 1980.
2. Signoret, J.-L. et al.: Aphasie sans amusie chez un organiste aveugle. *Rev Neurol (Paris)* **143, n° 3**, 1987.

CHAPTER 6

THE DYNAMICS OF SPEECH THERAPY IN APHASIA

C. CYR-STAFFORD

I believe that this difficulty is caused by certain humours. We, in our circle of wise men, call them deleterious humours (...) These are precisely what have brought on the muteness in your daughter.

Molière, *Le médecin malgré lui*

THE PLACE OF THE SPEECH THERAPY RELATIONSHIP IN THE HEALTH-CARE WORLD

To date, there has been little attention devoted to the study of the therapeutic relationship in clinical aphasiology. In a recent work, Ducarne de Ribaucourt[4] wrote that the relationship between the speech pathologist and the patient has never been described in detail or compared with other therapeutic relationships. In effect, that is precisely the aim of this chapter. As we shall discover, the relationship is multidimensional, and the notion of interpersonal dynamics can justifiably be applied to the relationship between the person with aphasia and the speech pathologist.

Just as aphasiology lies at the crossroads between neurology, linguistics, and psychology, the patient-speech pathologist relationship is akin to that of the doctor-patient, the student-teacher, and the therapist-client. Like doctors and teachers, speech pathologists possess unique knowledge. Like psychologists, they use their know-how and life-experience to help patients.

The common ground between the rehabilitation and the pedagogical relationships has a relatively long duration and an academic regularity. However, appearances are deceiving and one should avoid jumping to conclusions as to the inherent similarity between pedagogical and therapeutic relationships. In fact, the objective of speech therapy is not to learn something new but rather to reactivate inhibited abilities, to reorganize residual skills, or to develop compensatory strategies. It is the speech pathologist's duty to explain these differences to the patient.

As in psychotherapy, the speech pathologist-client relationship in aphasia centers around communication. When the communication deficit is so severe that it prevents necessary psychological intervention, the therapist will most effectively provide support and assistance in manageable doses during daily treatment sessions.

The history of medicine teaches us that, before we entered the consumer age, doctors were considered so omniscient that their presence alone was often sufficient to cure patients. This legacy of magical power was reinforced, over the last century, by the social and economic prestige that characterized the medical profession. According to Valabrega[14], physicians' prestige is closely linked to their contact with death, and reaches its apex in surgeons, whose practice mimics death and resurrection.

Whereas sorcerers cured by expelling illness and transferring it to external sources such as voodoo dolls, modern medicine and science have evolved to the point that the practitioners virtually ignore the patient, and uniquely focus on the disease. In an effort by Balint[1] to reverse the swing of the pendulum, the doctor-patient relationship has been analyzed in depth. The effectiveness of medical intervention was called into question by the works of Illitch[8], and the economic costs were criticized mercilessly. Then apparently an equilibrium was reached. In the late 1970s, Escande wrote:

"Like chess, medicine requires two players: There can be no good medicine if the population is not educated, if it is not explained what a doctor is, and how to make use of this great priest who is also a servant, and a jack-of-all-trades, who is asked to play each of these roles in turn."[6]

More recently, Coërs reminded his colleagues that:

> "We can improve an unhealthy situation by the mere fact of making it more comprehensible — by inciting in the patient the desire to actively participate in the domination and control over the course of his recovery."[2]

How do speech pathologists fit into this scenario? Like doctors, speech pathologists possess expertise. They too are filled with the fervent desire to cure. In addition, they appear to be gifted with magical powers when they can produce speech in a person with aphasia who "could not speak any more." The therapists' power, however, is relatively modest. Some doubt the specificity of speech pathologists' knowledge. Every speaking adult claims to understand the nature of language since he can speak so effortlessly. Non-specialists' efforts to assist persons with aphasia are usually ineffectual. At best, they hinder the ongoing speech therapy, and, in the worst cases, they impede the patient's development at an optimal period for therapy. The speech pathologists' power is also limited by their place at the bottom of the health-care hierarchy. There is always someone in a higher position who counsels patients not to worry, that the problem will take care of itself, or that the speech pathologist will solve everything. Finally, as opposed to the doctor, who can retreat from the mourning process, the speech pathologist must accompany persons with aphasia as they pass through the mourning stages that are associated with the loss of or changes to communicative abilities. Furthermore, they must simultaneously motivate patients to strive towards recovering their lost language skills.

THE THERAPEUTIC RELATIONSHIP AND THE THERAPY CONTRACT

Notwithstanding its therapeutic aspects, in aphasia the therapist-client relationship should be viewed, above all, as an encounter between two different individuals. These two adults differ not only in their personal experience, but also in their status in the present situation. Who is the person with aphasia? An individual in mourning. Who is the speech pathologist? An alleged wizard. Despite these differences in life story, personality, and status, the two must share the experience of a therapeutic relationship that requires both confidence and motivation.

Coërs's recommendation to doctors is fundamental to the relationship between the speech pathologist and the person with aphasia. Medicine can be administered to a passive subject, the limbs of an unconscious patient can be passively stimulated, but communication cannot be reestablished passively. The therapeutic relationship in aphasia requires that the client participate in decision-making, a measure known as the therapy contract. The main clauses of this contract revolve around counselling and joint agreement on decisions at all stages of treatment: evaluation, diagnosis, reeducation, rehabilitation, termination, and reintegration into the family, society, or into an institution. Just as each new specialist must forge a new therapeutic relationship, the professional must, from the first meeting, discuss the therapy contract, and reassess it with each major decision.

The therapeutic relationship responds to the needs of a human being who is undergoing a difficult and traumatic period which may have severe repercussions. In contrast, the therapy contract is based on scientific data. The literature contains cases of global aphasia, where the patients are trapped without communication, and, at the other end of the spectrum, cases of spontaneous recovery. Each year there is increasing evidence of the effectiveness of speech therapy in the treatment of aphasia. Although the following hypothesis cannot be easily supported, it seems that it is only under certain conditions affected by the degree, duration, start of treatment and the use of the most effective therapeutic approach that speech therapy produces results that are superior to other forms of treatment. The speech pathologist must share these findings with the patient.

The therapeutic relationship and the therapy contract should not be measured by the same criteria. The first type of relationship is one of assistance, and the help the patient receives is not quantifiable. How can the worth or the efficacy of a smile, encouragement, or a repeated explanation be measured? Note that from the start, the decision to commence treatment is made in conjunction with the person with aphasia. The illness and hospitalization can cause patients to feel that they have lost control over their lives — a dehumanizing experience. By giving the persons with aphasia some degree of control, speech therapy also grants them a certain dignity. From the moment that re-education starts to demand effort and work, it becomes essential that the investment be profitable for both the person with aphasia and the speech pathologist. In countries where speech therapy is practiced in a free market economy, without government intervention, the contract is an essential element of the therapeutic relationship. Both parties agree on an evaluation and a given number of sessions, thus clearly stipulating the objectives and financial outlay required. The contract will only be reviewed following a reassessment and a sharing of information. In this context, the sharing of the decision-making is evident: Both parties will decide when to terminate, pursue, or alter the course of treatment.

In our view, spoon-feeding should play no part in the dynamics of the speech therapy relationship. On the contrary, the relationship should support and foster maximal autonomy for persons with aphasia as they strive to cope with aphasia. The role of the speech pathologist is that of a companion who provides unconditional encouragement. If, as some philosophers claim, language is the essence of humankind, then aphasia, since it strikes a person's very being, can and should only belong to the person who acquires the syndrome.

TRUST

The therapeutic relationship or contract can only be developed in an atmosphere of trust. Plunged into a new situation, persons with aphasia who have not yet had an unpleasant experience or acquired a poor outlook, will naturally place all their trust in the person who offers to help them and to explain the nature of their communication problems. As a health-care professional, the speech pathologist benefits from the esteem that is generally displayed towards health-care professionals. The respect granted to doctors trickles down, in effect, to the speech pathologist. To truly gain the patient's trust, however, therapists must prove their competence.

Alongside the *knowledge* that the speech pathologist offers to share are the know-how and experience that will play a major role in establishing and maintaining trusting relationships. The know-how used may vary widely according to the stage of treatment, and the type and severity of aphasia. The experience essentially involves professional qualities. Most persons with aphasia and their families will quickly learn that speech therapy requires *patience*. It is obvious that both the speech pathologist and the client must take the time to get acquainted and to establish communication channels.

The serene attitude of the knowledgeable professional who is familiar with these situations is reassuring to the person with aphasia.

Serenity does not imply indifference, however, since an indifferent approach will cause the patient to feel like an object. The aphasia therapist must convey *empathy* and *concern* not only verbally, but also by means of gestures, looks, and listening techniques. *Intellectual honesty* is another basic quality and an essential ingredient in the trusting relationship cocktail. A patient who senses hidden motivations will tend to distrust the therapist. Persons with aphasia believe that they are disabled and profoundly diminished. This feeling creates negative attitudes that Tanner and Gerstenberger[13] liken to the classic stages of mourning. The speech pathologist should tolerate these responses without making value judgments. Denial should be anticipated: Persons with aphasia may disagree with the diagnosis or attribute the communication problem to the listener. They may retreat into *passivity* while waiting for a miracle or hope that their will to recover will suffice to cure them. *Frustration* and *aggression* are other common reactions. Speech pathologists must allow the patients to vent their anger and must not allow themselves to be *manipulated.* Aphasia therapists will inevitably face a patient's *depression;* this should be considered a natural reaction to the realization of a loss that, we stress, affects the very essence of the human being.

In the midst of this emotional turmoil, the person needs the unconditional acceptance which the speech pathologist offers. This is where *compassion* is manifested in the speech pathologist-client relationship. In conclusion, we wish to emphasize that the trusting relationship seems to be eminently subtle and cultural, and we are aware that we are only skimming the surface in this description.

MOTIVATION

Love and hate are known to be compelling sources of motivation; these feelings, however, are not inherent in therapeutic relationships. Respect for authority can also stimulate a desire to "follow the doctor's orders," but aphasia rehabilitation is much more demanding. At any rate, this prestige has no role to play in authentic communication — an essential element of speech therapy. How can the person, anosognosic, or overcome by what Lubinsky[10] calls the "crisis of aphasia," possibly find the motivation that is needed for therapy? Though trust can be gained from the start, the same cannot be said for motivation. Some patients deny their condition, others are convinced that it is transitory. Still others engage in wishful thinking. Clearly, awareness of one's disability and reactional depression do little to foster motivation. Here too, the speech pathologist plays a crucial role since motivation will be contingent on the quality of the interpersonal relationship. The therapy contract arising from an objective assessment is yet another factor that strengthens motivation.

Motivation theory suggests that motivation is based on the *hope* of reaching certain levels of satisfaction. Such theories also assert that *needs* are hierarchically *ordered;* food and shelter are primal needs, while professional success is on another level of satisfaction. Between the state of *dissatisfaction* that produces motivation, and the state of *satisfaction,* lies an intermediary state of *non-dissatisfaction* that saps motivation. Two other elements detract from or stimulate motivation: the *probability* of achieving satisfaction, and the amount of effort required, with its corollary — individual aptitudes.

How do these notions borrowed from industrial psychology shed light on the patient's motivation in aphasia rehabilitation? For example, on what level is the communication suppressed by aphasia situated? In some cases, it is on the primary level of expression of psychological needs. In others, it is the social isolation created by slow and laborious communication or the disregard for social conventions in conversation. Anosognosia and motivation are therefore contradictory. In cases of anosognosia, the patient will only submit to examinations and rehabilitation sessions in order to comply with or please the therapist.

Persons with aphasia can achieve satisfaction solely through the complete recovery of language. It is only when they can communicate "like before" that this state will be reached. Recovery from aphasia depends, in part, on the energy invested in rehabilitation; the effort is proportional to the hopes for recovery. Rehabilitation only implies a possible improvement, without issuing guarantees or nourishing false hopes. It is clearly difficult to stimulate motivation towards what is merely a potential lessening of dissatisfaction. Realistically, the object of re-education can only be non-dissatisfaction. Out of hundreds of cases, we have never witnessed a single patient who was completely satisfied with his language performance. Even when tests reveal only residual symptoms, the person with aphasia no longer experiences the joys of conversation, reading, and speaking "like before."

For persons with aphasia, individual aptitudes correspond to the residual abilities outlined in Wepman's model, today known as the potential for improvement. Here again, the speech pathologist plays a crucial role. He or she must explain the results of the assessment, and clarify the improvements (often fine and imperceptible to the patient), which were achieved through stimulation, simplification, or alternate procedures. The therapist must also specify the degree of effort required. He or she should restrain the enthusiast who requests six hours of speech therapy daily so that he can recover sooner, or to remind a discouraged patient of the progress since the previous or initial evaluation. He or she should explain that mastering oral language requires several years, and recovering written language, a few more. Speech pathologists are walking on a tightrope when they discuss the possibility of the patient attaining his goal: To speak like before. Gradually, the patient will be made to realize that this idealistic aim will fade over time, and that the energy he must invest in therapy can only bring about an improvement, or a decrease in dissatisfaction.

From the arguments above, we can conclude that motivation is contingent on several factors, and varies between people and situations. In the case of persons with aphasia, the determining factors are the characteristics of the type of aphasia and the time since the onset of the illness that treatment is initiated.

THE NATURE OF APHASIA

The type of aphasia also influences the therapeutic relationship since a patient who speaks little or not at all can gain confidence and motivation from the attention that the speech pathologist bestows as she patiently listens to his impoverished verbal performance. Through various strategies, the therapist enables the patient to improve his communication, and explains the absence of a certain word or a distorted sound. Trust and motivation are thus fostered by these initial attempts at authentic communication. Other health-care professionals who treat *persons with Broca's aphasia* often do not have the time to listen; furthermore, they are not qualified to help the patient. In this case the patient may wish the speech pathologist to become his spokesperson. The therapist must be tactful in order to cope with this delicate role, which is even more precarious to get out of than to take on. The specialist who can verbalize the patient's frustration will gain his confidence; the speech pathologist who becomes a translator, or messenger, risks creating a dependency which will ultimately limit motivation.

The needs of the *patient with Wernicke's aphasia,* e.g. a person whose comprehension is deficient and who often talks poorly and excessively, are quite different. A trusting relationship will be established most often through non-verbal communication. Of utmost importance is to explain to the person with Wernicke's aphasia that he is not "crazy." The problem treating these persons is that trust and motivation cannot be expressed verbally; unfortunately, the person often does not comprehend speech. Once the basic message:"I want to try to help you" has been conveyed, a demonstration must follow soon after. In fact, the patient with jargon aphasia who cannot comprehend must blindly trust in the therapist. Persons with Wernicke's aphasia respond well to objective measures. Take the time to repeat messages, use numerous strategies to aid comprehension (written and oral words, drawings, gestures), demand the patient's attention, but do so with humor. In other words, do anything that will work. The therapeutic relationship with the person with receptive defects is apparently more complex and admittedly more difficult. Therapy is more effective in cases where a trusted family member or friend of the patient enlists the therapist's help. Patients are more likely to respond to treatment when they agree to discard the mask and admit that they cannot understand.

Patients with global aphasia can best be treated with the help of someone who is emotionally close to them (a friend or relative). This person will speak for, as well as represent, the patient. He or she will be given all the information in the patient's presence, and will be involved in the negotiation of the therapy contract. Out of love for that family member or friend, the person with aphasia will persevere in improving his communication skills and will not become discouraged by setbacks. Without this important link, the required trust and motivation may give way to scepticism, defeatism, and passivity. If therapy does not bring about improvements in comprehension, expression, and written communication, the therapist will attempt to initiate compensatory mechanisms by enlisting the help of the spokesperson.

As seen above, the *severity* of the disability affects the therapeutic relationship. The interdependency between the potential level of autonomy and the severity of the communication deficit is quite observable. Even in cases of severe aphasia, the goal should be to maximize the patient's autonomy. This implies that persons with aphasia should never be excluded from discussions involving them. We know that comprehension is never completely nil, and that the pragmatic, emotional, and redundant features of language, which contribute to the complexity of communication, can spark flashes of comprehension in persons with aphasia.

PHASES OF TREATMENT

The person with aphasia and the speech pathologist meet not only at a precise moment in their personal history, but also at a point in the course of the aphasia. The therapeutic relationship must take this fact into account and adjust itself accordingly.

The Initial Phase

In this acute phase more than in those that follow, the therapeutic relationship can be likened to a balancing act. The persons with aphasia are being treated by various health-care professionals, primarily their doctor. They can easily meet thirty or more health-care workers during a short stay in a typical North American hospital. Therefore, the speech pathologist must stake her claim as soon as possible, ideally when the patient is still in the emergency ward.

According to Northouse[12], at this stage the relationship between the care-giver and the patient is more important than the actual message conveyed. The presence of the speech pathologist who diagnoses the aphasia and provides information is reassuring to the person with aphasia. For the time being, it is enough to observe the patient and determine the best moment for the assessment, which, the therapist should keep in mind, will probably be marked by defensive responses. The speech pathologist should aim towards preserving authentic communication at all costs, as it is not only the object of treatment, but also the essential link between the speech pathologist and the patient. The sharing of knowledge and decisions should begin at this point. The patient should be informed of the possibility of spontaneous recovery, and that sometimes treatment, e.g re-education, is required. If so, an objective assessment should be performed to examine the various aspects of language. At this point it would be cruel to mention failures in re-education, yet exaggerated optimism is a potential time bomb. It is too soon to doubt — now is the time for hope and the forging of the therapeutic relationship. The therapist must walk the line between scepticism and credulity. "I think" or "I don't think" should be replaced by "I don't know." At this point there is no certitude, just probabilities.

The Assessment

Every experienced speech pathologist can vouch for the value of an objective examination. In addition, they are well aware of the length of an examination that purports to cover the various aspects of language and functional communication. How can the patient with aphasia be prevented from erecting defense mechanisms along the way? With a therapy contract that stresses the importance of the evaluation of deficits and residual capacities so that a "made to order" treatment can be applied and progress can be measured. Although the assessment is objective, this should by no means deter the speech pathologist from helping the patient with each stage of the evaluation: If the first attempt fails, the patient can always try again using one of a panoply of assistance techniques. The examination is more precise because it reveals not only the success rate, but also attests to the range of means that facilitate the patient's performance. Moreover, it will be subsequently easier to chart the patient's progress. Conscientious speech pathologists reassess patients often. In a productive therapeutic relationship, by means of a series of examinations, one can observe the person with aphasia evolving from defensiveness to trust.

Re-education

As soon as the evaluation is complete, the speech pathologist discusses the results with the person and plans the objectives of re-education. At this point, as discussed by Howard and Hatfield[7], the therapeutic program can focus on restoration or reconstitution of the lost functions. In the first case, the function is reestablished to its level prior to the illness. In the second case, through the use of other strategies, the patient can reach comparable proficiency despite a definitive loss. Either way, the progression of treatment should be strict and ordered; in no event should stages be skipped, or the therapy rushed. As the classics dictate, the starting point is success, but the objective revolves around deficits and improvement. The task can be considered to be shared: the speech pathologist points the way, the person with aphasia follows. Independent efforts, outside of therapy, will enable persons with aphasia to fulfil their role in the therapeutic process. This almost always painstaking work also creates frustrations that compound the ones initially induced by the language deficit. Depressive reactions often surface and cloud the re-education period. The speech pathologist must constantly refocus the therapeutic relationship on the task at hand, while being attentive, highly receptive, and tolerant towards the display of emotional problems. Once again, the aphasia therapist is performing a balancing act between scientific rigor and the needs of a real human being — a balance between efficacy and humanism.

Rehabilitation

Rehabilitation is yet another critical stage, one where patients must admit that they will never again be "like before." The helping relationship predominates at this point. The re-education strategy now revolves around compensation. Over the short or long run, the patient will reach a plateau. Compensation can be accomplished by using other modalities of language or by resorting to gestures or drawings — an option that some consider repulsive. Anthropology holds that through the course of phylogenetic evolution, by speaking, humans freed their hands so that they could use tools. Communication subsequently became more effective and more economical. It is quite normal that compensatory mechanisms which are only *ersatz* forms of language will be reluctantly accepted by the patient, who will founder in grief for the loss of language. Aside from participating in rehabilitation per se, which aims to maximize performance despite the communication deficits, therapists must also support patients until they accept their condition. In fact, this is the ultimate goal of rehabilitation: To bring about acceptance in persons with aphasia of their loss of language and to allow them to dissociate their personal identity from their present condition as a speaker or listener.

Separation, Termination, and Group Interaction

The termination of treatment will be less stressful if the therapy contract was clearly defined, discussed, and amended throughout the previous phases of therapy. The reaction to separation will be milder if, along with a decrease in intensity of treatment, the therapist encourages social reintegration through self-help or therapy groups. This orientation will also enable the patient to share with peers any apprehension regarding the termination of treatment. Finally, it is easier to join associations or support groups if one is already acquainted with another person with aphasia. Naturally, the same principle applies for small groups of patients.

In this final stage, therapists should analyze with the persons with aphasia the impact and significance of aphasia on their personal life. Some find that their work is affected, others are concerned about their social lives. Speech pathologists should act as intermediaries as much as possible. They will help the patient to place the impact of aphasia into perspective by making analogies to the hearing-impaired, to foreign tourists, and to those who speak freely in dictatorial regimes — all people whose communication is impaired. If the relationship is not terminated abruptly, the speech pathologist may reap the rewards of hearing the person joke, or hearing a group of persons with aphasia bursting into laughter.

THE ENLARGED DYAD

The currents that characterize the therapeutic relationship flow between two people: The speech pathologist and the person with aphasia. Dependence may subsequently ensue if the therapist is endowed with the dual role of official spokesperson and privileged conversation partner. Although a clear therapy contract helps to avoid this pitfall, it does not solve the problem of generalizing the patient's abilities. In our department, the experience of sharing patients is a necessity due to the part-time status of many speech pathologists. As a result, we have observed a dual level of performance by the person with aphasia in relation to the chief speech pathologist (the person responsible for the patient's file, evaluation, and the progress of therapy) and the associate. One of the objectives of the reeducation/rehabilitation phase is therefore to generalize maximal communication with another specialist. This procedure has proven to be beneficial and has spread throughout the clinic. Currently, persons with aphasia are systematically treated by two specialists.

The participation of the person with aphasia in group therapy, directed by speech pathologists who are not necessarily those who treat the patients on an individual basis, is another effective method of expanding the helping relationship and enabling patients to generalize their communicative skills.

CONCLUSION

We would like to conclude with the following observation by Marshall[11]: "One does not become an aphasia clinician overnight. To become an aphasia clinician, one must see many persons with aphasia over a prolonged period of time. This accomplishment demands study, observation and thought. While it is possible to learn about aphasia in the classroom, from reading the literature and observing in the laboratory, it is impossible to learn much more about aphasic people without spending a significant time in what Jay Rosenbek (1984) has called 'the clinical trenches.'"

REFERENCES

1. Balint, M.: *Le médecin, son malade et la maladie*, P.U.F., Paris, 1960.
2. Coërs, C.: *Médecins ou magiciens. Mythologie de l'art de guérir*, Arthaud, Paris, 1985.
3. Cyr-Stafford, C.: Recovery of auditory comprehension in aphasia: Is language therapy effective? *Journal of Neurolinguistics,* **2, n° 1,** 1986.
4. Ducarne de Ribaucourt, B.:*Rééducation sémiologique de l'aphasie,* Masson, Paris, 1986.
5. Escande, J.-P.: *Les médecins,* Grasset, Paris, 1975.
6. Escande, J.-P.: *Les malades*, Grasset, Paris, 1977.
7. Howard, D. & F.M. Hatfield: *Aphasia Therapy: Historical and Contemporary Issues,* Erlbaum, London, 1987.
8. Illitch, Y.: *Némésis médicale*, Seuil, Paris, 1975.
9. Joanette, Y. et al.: Intervention orthophonique auprès des aphasiques, **in** *Neuropsychologie clinique et neurologie du comportement.* Botez, M.-I., P.U.M. & Masson, Montreal & Paris, 1987.
10. Lubinsky, R.: Environmental Language Intervention, **in** *Language Intervention Strategies in Adult Aphasia,* Chapey, R., Williams & Wilkins, Baltimore, 1981.
11. Marshall, R.C.: *Case Studies in Aphasia Rehabilitation: For Clinicians by Clinicians,* Pro-Ed, Austin, 1986.
12. Northouse, P.G. & L.L. Northouse: *Health Communication,* Prentice-Hall, Englewood-Cliffs, 1985.
13. Tanner, D.C. & D.L. Gerstenberger: The Grief Response in Neuropathologies of Speech and Language, *Aphasiology,* **2, n° 1,** 1988.
14. Valabrega, J.-P.: *La relation thérapeutique malade et médecin,* Flammarion, Médecine-Sciences, Paris, 1962.

Chapter 7

TYPICAL BEHAVIOR OF PERSONS WITH APHASIA AND THEIR FAMILIES

J. PONZIO AND R. DEGIOVANI

The average of a series of inexact measurements does not necessarily lead to a correct assessment.

Waters

The problem of the subject with aphasia remains the same. Nothing is resolved, everything becomes more acute, and there are fewer means to combat the problem.

Serge Zlatine

INTRODUCTION

In this chapter we will examine a series of behavioral types that can be observed in persons with aphasia, as well as the corresponding structures in the person's family.

The study below, inspired by natural history, does not claim to be neurolinguistic or medical. In fact, it resembles more closely a sociological or literary description, similar to the one found in La Bruyère.

Within the family unit, the person with aphasia is quickly branded a patient; he must battle not only with his language problem, but also with common misconceptions about the nature of his disability: "Doctor, he understands everything." These misconceptions arise from principles of the psychology of the individual and especially mechanisms of family structure. Faced with aphasia, family members may exhibit catastrophic reactions, rejection, or even the opposite — overprotection, and occasionally outright denial of the illness. If these responses, which are often manifested simultaneously, are not taken into account, they may be detrimental to therapy.

THE PERSON WITH APHASIA

Total Invalid or Infantilized Martyr

For the time being, we shall not dwell on these first two categories; they will appear below in the discussion of overprotective families. Everyone knows examples of people who are completely dependent, unable to perform even the simplest everyday task; who do not get up from their wheelchairs even once they are capable of standing as well as walking.

Also on record are accounts of infantilized martyrs whose families, not always motivated by ill-will, forbid them to engage in any voluntary movement or activity, turn away visitors, downplay the value of medical attention and are even more strongly opposed to speech therapy.

In fact, these two *types,* the invalid and the martyr, are two sides of the same coin, depending on whether the passivity originates within the patient or within the family context.

The Apathetic Outcast and the Nobel Prize Winner

Some patients experience minimal residual symptoms. They are neither paralyzed nor impaired in either hearing or speech. Acceptable communication is still within their means. Perhaps they have residual dysarthria or a subtle comprehension deficit, the only sign that at one point there was a breakdown — something wrong inside them. In this case, the language deficit is induced by a lesion in the brain, the problem is resolved in rehabilitation, and the person recovers, yet the difficulties linger on!

Despite the speech pathologist's efforts, the psychologist's care, and regular consultations with the doctor, these persons with aphasia possess, or will eventually recover, a faculty which they fail to use! For example, the wife of Philip, a person with aphasia, has joined an association for persons with aphasia while her husband spent his time in bars, guzzling beer!

The Nobel Prize for Rehabilitation is another example of neglected residual language abilities. The person with aphasia, willing, industrious, and devoted, is capable of impressive demonstrations of his/her language abilities under examination or when in the presence of the single most favorite speech pathologist. Word-finding difficulties are minor or moderate, paraphasias are scarce or nonexistent, dysarthria is residual, and comprehension is adequate. *The patient can be made to say whatever you want.* As far as the patients are concerned, even though they have been successfully rehabilitated, they cannot or will not speak or express their thoughts by means of language. Outside of the therapy context they do not talk, they only do exercises. They are like performers who simply practice scales. Although they do not attempt to communicate through speech, they are quite capable of speaking.

This dichotomy between the faculty and its use, between theoretical competence and practical performance, can be described in terms of the opposition between severity and acuteness: The severity of the basic neurolinguistic disturbance, and the acuteness of the impairment to language use. The two parameters are usually fairly proportional one to the other. In the Nobel Prize winner, the gap between severity and acuteness is extreme. The severity revealed by testing is minimal, but extreme acuteness is present in situations involving communication. These patients are usually the most noble failures of speech therapy. They put forth a tremendous amount of effort to win the Nobel Prize; however, this effort is for all intents and purposes in vain. Fortunately, this status is usually temporary.

This description of the various stereotypes is by no means exhaustive. These character types should be considered both individually as well as within their family environment. At any rate, rehabilitation, in general, is best approached systemically, similar to the methods used in families where no organic disorder exists. In cases where the organic pathology is manifested by an acquired language disorder, persons with aphasia cannot be artificially extracted from their family environment, any more than a fish can be observed outside its aquarium.

The fact that families may respond to, exclude, avoid or distress the person with aphasia obviously complicates the issue, which should be a joint concern of both client and therapist.

THE FAMILIES OF PERSONS WITH APHASIA

> *The human race is characterized by a singular development of social relations that supports the exceptional capacities of mental communication, and, in correlation, by a paradoxical economy of instinct that reveal themselves to be basically susceptible to conversion and inversion and can only be sporadically isolated. Thus an infinite variety of adaptive behaviors is possible... This dimension characterizes the family, as do all social phenomena in humanity.*
>
> Jacques Lacan

In the second half of this chapter, we propose a description of a few family types of persons with aphasia. This categorization borrows equally from natural history and the game "Sept Familles,"[1] and clearly does not claim to be scientific. The examples below are presented because they do exist and are models to be avoided if possible. They should be considered as pathological forms of family dynamics which are reflected in the interaction between the person with aphasia and other family members. By *pathological,* we are referring to the outer limits of *normality,* which can be conceptualized as though forces within society were repelling the pathological behavior.

---

[1] Seven families is a card game played by children in France. In this game, players must, either by drawing cards or asking each other, get face cards which can form whole families.

The goal here is certainly not to confine the person with aphasia and his family to a rigid classification which is neither exhaustive nor of any proven value. Nonetheless, these outlines, occasionally caricature-like, should allow health-care professionals and family members of persons with aphasia to more clearly perceive the modes of communication that may surface between them, and to request psychological assistance when needed. Perhaps the elucidation of diverse family relations will be potentially useful in the therapeutic context from which it stems.

States of Non-communication

Nobody home...

If a group does not consider itself as such, it is not due to an individual or collective absence of thought. Lack of communication within a family is not a situation limited to groups where one of the members has a specific verbal impairment. That would be too simple! Group communication characterized by a lack of emotion and which serves mainly as commentary is called *empty speech*. Yet if one of the members of the group loses the ability to speak, then problems related to the disturbance of communication within the family may surface which would not have been manifested otherwise.

In this scenario, only outsiders will be able to pinpoint the root of the problem and subsequently to propose a solution. Yet in such cases of *group foolishness,* there is often no request for assistance of this nature. As a speech therapist, one can and often must ask oneself "Why treat such a person?" A person is not necessarily more excluded from the group that does not consider itself as such; the group will tend less to consider the person as a foreign body to be absorbed or rejected. The person is just there, like a pet, or a picture on the wall. Pets are fed, and their litter baskets are changed occasionally; likewise, picture frames are dusted once a month — the obligation ends there.

The therapist must be a diehard meddler to want to modify a system that is so well-balanced, a *status quo* where there is no otherness, difference, and possibly even no suffering... But the speech therapist who permeates this group, either through professional connections, neighborly relations, chance, or any other means, introduces, by his presence alone, a need for reconsideration. Before any action is taken, there is a destabilization that, in most cases, tends to decrease and ultimately stop on its own. Nonetheless, this common spontaneous reaction does not preclude reflection on the effects of the therapist's presence.

Apparently, the foremost quality of a therapist, overall, but especially in this context, is humility: The ability to admit that things can only be as they are. If the patient can again comment on, or at least revel an interest in television shows; if he can participate in lottery drawings, and can laugh or cry along with everyone else, then these are the humble objectives which the therapist should accept.

Indifference

Keep talking, I'm listening.

The following situation is similar enough to the previous example for it to be presented immediately after, but different enough to justify its own heading. This scenario is often a facade, behind which is concealed a potent dose of hatred; hatred which was suppressed before the stroke, and could no longer be expressed afterwards — you do not kick a man when he is down.

The family admits but ignores the fact that the person with aphasia can think and desire on his own. Here, some of the most dramatic situations can be observed: Outright denial of everything that can be considered a vital need of an individual, i.e. the total absence of recognition of the person's desperate attempts at communication.

As for the satisfaction of vital needs, the need to communicate is surely primordial. For example, speech that is labored or erroneous may still convey meaning, the meaning must be correctly interpreted and produce the desired effect. During this stage, persons with aphasia often have a keener appreciation of the intricacies of family life; they intuitively understand much better the motivations behind family members' behavior. Unfortunately, their opinions no longer count. The new situation created by their unemployment also implies that they are now housebound and can offer input into domestic issues more than they did before the illness. Now, however, no one listens, and their words fall on deaf ears.

Of course, it is unthinkable to deprive the person of his basic needs such as food, elimination, and sexual functions. The satisfaction of these needs, however, will often be the grounds for countless retaliations for those who were previously snubbed, since the family now has complete control over when and where these needs will be satisfied. They zealously enforce strict compliance with schedules, settings, and outings. The absoluteness of these rules is often more apparent than their necessity.

In this context, the satisfaction of the sexual needs of the person with aphasia is simply inconceivable. The spouse will often provide numerous excuses or deny that the person with aphasia has sexual urges: "In his condition, doctor, I wouldn't dream of it!" As in other aspects of everyday life, this condition often becomes even more acute if the person with aphasia is female. She may even find herself alone, divorced or separated, thanks to her spouse and the legal system. Suicide is sometimes the last assertion of her existence. Psychological intervention is not an option — another fine opportunity for revenge! Even speech therapy is often scoffed at, and the results are downplayed. The person's doctor is thus obliged to accept a situation where there is no hope of progress. He will ultimately cease to recommend speech therapy which has become futile.

Rejection

Get out of my Life, Damn You!

Exclusion is sometimes the fate of the person with aphasia when the family's attitudes are characterized by indifference. This exclusion, however, may be considerably more obvious in cases where it constitutes the only symptom. Note that exclusion is not one-sided. The exclusion of someone from the normal functioning of a group can be manifested through radical means, i.e., assassination. Of course this is an extreme case, but it occurs nonetheless. Other forms of exclusion are more subtle and also more socially acceptable. Exclusion can be physical or spiritual, disappearance in the eyes of the law or symbolic murder.

If we briefly reflect on the means of damning a person with aphasia or any other patient to purgatory, we can appreciate the extreme convenience of the various care institutions which have sprung up in modern societies. Admittedly, people find it difficult actively to commit their parents to institutions. In fact many long stays are absolutely justified, even necessitated, by the persons' condition, especially if their chances of rehabilitation are slim. Nonetheless, in the Western world, pages and pages of professional directories are filled with a wide variety of institutions that cater to all types of patients. The advertisements praise the merits of one home or another, all with the most qualified staff, outstanding care facilities, and a utopian atmosphere. Evidently, the existence of institutions where one can place one's sick relative for long, sometimes very prolonged, stays corresponds to a social need as much as it does a strictly medical one. Meanwhile, it may even be the case that some of these homes do not have the most qualified staff, outstanding care facilities, and a utopian atmosphere!

Symbolic exclusion, less drastic and not immediately obvious, can still be undeniably as effective. For example, each decision, from the most insignificant one to the one that concerns the person with aphasia the most, is made without the individual's knowledge or without direct consultation. Other decisions are reached despite awareness of the person's opposition, either as it was formerly stated or expressed using his residual speaking skills. In these cases, the person is a victim of violence, through exclusion which bears a strong resemblance to assassination! In this respect, society shrugs its shoulders. Better yet, society has provided perverse safety measures which aggravate the situation. Although these measures were introduced to protect persons and property from themselves and from others, they are sometimes used as a means of exclusion. Legal protection excludes persons with aphasia from most of the decisions regarding themselves. The legal system can work to the persons' disadvantage, and can even be used to demonstrate to others the severity of the disability, the acuteness of the impairments, and why not the self-sacrifice of the spouse, who milks the legal aspects of the context for his or her own glory...

The Smotherers

Poor You!

Very often, the family's attitude towards the person with aphasia seems acceptable to outsiders: There is no visible cruelty, indifference, or rejection. Instead, the person with aphasia is cajoled, pampered, his speech and needs are anticipated, and the words are practically taken right out of his mouth. To want to speak... The use of language remains, in these people as in children, inseparable from individual autonomy. Like the small child whose overly-attentive supervision will prevent development and maturing into an independent adult, the person with aphasia is constantly *protected* from any external harm, including... the one posed by speech therapy and the efforts it demands. At this point, the wife of the person with aphasia (most often, but not exclusively) has a prime opportunity to reassume her maternal role as an overprotective mother hen. To this type of victim of familial overprotection, we have given the names *total invalid and infantilized martyr.*

This type of family relation is interesting because of the decoding that it requires. In this case, the discernment of the existential reality of the group is impossible to achieve if one relies on the evident signs: Demonstrations or claims of love bestowed on the person with aphasia by the spouse. The denial of reality that underlies this type of scenario is actually more authentic than all the superficial vows. In other words, one must always seek the truth which lies behind these masks and must strive to gain a clear perception of family relations as if one were looking through a prism that inverts objects into a mirror image of what meets the eye.

In all fairness, definitive family consensus and tacit or explicit agreement among all family members must always incite therapists to seek the real reasons behind this unanimity. To admit that the main reason for this pity is to disguise an imponderable aggression is, here, at least as close to the truth as believing, or pretending to believe, the saintly attitude manifested through good will: "Oh! If it wasn't for me, what would become of you?"

The Spectacular Feat

He can say whatever you want

This person with aphasia, who performs so well in therapy, as he does within the family, is an important person. Doubtless, this was true before the illness. In this setting he retains his prestige. But his worth as a person with aphasia can only be measured if it affects the entire group, who find in it a justification for their existence and their cohesion.

The attentive family quickly learns all the facilitation techniques: Automatic series, sentence completion, oral and semantic cues, recitations, prayers, and songs. They witness the miracle of the *mute who is made to speak,* and are mesmerized by appearances. Their fascination with the form of sounds prevents them from considering the independent thought of the patient. They are convinced that the only possible thought is expressible thought. Note that these efforts are often helpful to speech pathologists since they can indicate the future course of treatment, i.e. the way in which the person can use his evolving language capacities. That is why a family who functions on the basis of spectacular feats should never be criticized. These are almost always temporary attitudes that characterize a stage in the relationship with the rehabilitating person with aphasia. At a later stage it will be possible to spur the person towards the ideal: Spontaneous communication.

CONCLUSION

These assorted stereotypes of family structure correspond more or less with certain types of persons with aphasia described elsewhere. Therefore it is hardly useful, to avoid the word *fruitless,* to question whether the *primum movens* is found in patients or in their family. The structures which reveal exaggeration or pathological deviance AFTER the stroke, were all erected BEFORE, with the participation of the same individual who subsequently seems to be caught in the web that he himself helped spin. That is why the therapeutic approach, not to aphasia but to group pathology in general, should be inherently systemic. That is, it should take into account all the individuals who make up the group and should monitor their reciprocal psychological relations.

In cases where there is no love or request for assistance, it is the *superficial* intervention represented by speech therapy that can spark the recovery of the person's identity. In cases where hatred or aggression is present within the family, these feelings may be reoriented, and be consciously or unconsciously diverted. In cases where an excess of apparent love both hides and reveals real smothering, analytical psychotherapy can be quite beneficial.

Of course, in this particular context, the demand for assistance is not expressed, not only because it may not exist in all cases, but also because of the language impairment. It is therefore difficult to imagine how treatment can be successfully initiated in this situation.

REFERENCES

1. Ponzio, J.: Existe-t-il un sujet aphasique?, **in** *Actes du congrès scientifique international d'orthophonie,* l'Ortho-édition, Isbergues, France, 1987.

CHAPTER 8

THE BILINGUAL PERSON WITH APHASIA — THE AUSTRALIAN CONTEXT

A. WHITWORTH AND H. SJARDIN

The onset of aphasia confronts individuals and their families with a host of changes with which they need to come to terms. When the aphasic is bilingual, or multilingual, and often living within a different culture, additional issues to those facing the monolingual are raised for the individual, the family, and the service providers. This chapter will explore some of those issues for the aphasic whose native language is other than English with particular reference to the speech-language pathologist in Australia, a predominantly monolingual professional in an increasingly multicultural community. The relevance of such issues, however, extends beyond the Australian context. They are in essence common to every country, whether it be due to historical factors or to increasing population mobility. The histories of three bilingual aphasics who attended one Australian clinic are described followed by an exploration of the issues raised by each. Suggestions are made for possible strategies to overcome some of the difficulties facing the aphasic, the health professional, and society.

CASE STUDIES

Case Study 1

Mrs. W. is a 68 year old Dutch widow who, at the time of onset of aphasia, had been living in Australia for 23 years. When found collapsed at home, she was described as speaking only Dutch which was garbled and slurred. Previously, she was described as reasonably fluent in English but with a strong accent and some Dutch words interspersed. A diagnosis was made of moderate expressive aphasia in Dutch and severe expressive aphasia in English.

The speech-language pathologist working with Mrs. W. spoke both English and Dutch and was able to establish with formal assessment that skills such as naming, picture description, and reading were consistently superior in Dutch and that comprehension of both languages was relatively intact. Mrs. W. stated that she found Dutch easier to understand and speak. When speaking English she tended to confuse the two languages and often inappropriately spoke Dutch to an English-speaking person. She was mostly unaware when this occurred. This latter confusion did not occur when talking Dutch. Indeed, in the early stage of hospitalization, Mrs. W. reported increased "confusion" and disorientation when hearing English. Her level of understanding increased when information was clarified in Dutch. An illustration of the interference of Dutch when speaking English is seen below in the transcription of a picture description task using the picnic scene from the Western Aphasia Battery[12]. The Dutch words are underlined.

"There *is een boom een* car *een* man with *een* book, *een meisje, wat is dat een meisje — een vrouw, een* cool drink. *Ik zeg dat goed heh! Dat weet ik niet of ik dat doed zeg. De jongen zit* on the beach and he has a shovel *en een* dog on the beach."

Translated into English, this reads,

"There is a tree a car a man with a book, a girl, what is that a girl—a woman, a cool drink. I say that well eh! I don't know if I say that well. The boy sits on the beach and he has a shovel and a dog on the beach."

When Mrs. W. spoke Dutch, her language was more fluent and cohesive and there was little interference from English. While Mrs. W. was speaking English, there was no significant difference in the degree of language switching that occured when speaking to monolingual and bilingual English speakers. Her two sons spoke Dutch but not her daughter-in-law or grandchildren. She had a number of friends who spoke a mixture of English and Dutch. During her hospitalization, Mrs. W. talked of alienation from the hospital environment, loneliness, and her continuing grief related to her recently deceased husband.

Therapy was started initially in Dutch alone as it was the stated preferred language and less disordered. An important aim of therapy was to reduce confusion at both a general and a linguistic level. At the same time Mrs. W. was regularly reminded and encouraged to become aware of when she was speaking Dutch to English-speaking people. Once Dutch had improved in fluency it was considered appropriate to focus on therapy in English while continuing encouragement to separate clearly the two languages for different people and situations. As English was still important to use in her social environment, this could not be ignored. To maintain social support and the experience of easy and successful communication, interaction with pure Dutch-speaking friends was encouraged. This included facilitating contact with the Dutch Australian Society.

Unlike her monolingual English-speaking aphasic counterpart, Mrs. W. was confronted with a confusing and differential impairment of the two languages in which she had previously been fluent. The significant people in her life were both bi- and monolingual. However Mrs. W.'s ability to communicate with her family was initially limited to Dutch speakers, thereby isolating her from other family members and her English-speaking environment. Her tendency to "code switch" between the two languages and her inability to monitor this switching from one language to the other further reduced the success of her communication.

Likewise, the speech-language pathologist was faced with the dilemma of first identifying the relative degree of breakdown in the two languages and then making ongoing management decisions concerning the most appropriate language of intervention. Assessment tasks that tapped the intricacies of language and its breakdown needed to be both available and utilized by the speech-language pathologist who had a working knowledge of Dutch, a language spoken by only three percent of the Australian population[3]. To ensure an optimum intervention environment, it was essential to identify Mrs. W.'s language choice and the increased confusion that resulted for her when English was spoken. The particular ways in which language was used within the various facets of her social and family environment needed to be considered at all stages of Mrs. W.'s management. Encouraging a personalized social milieu to meet her emotional as well as language needs was an important facet of overall management.

Case Study 2

Mr. S. is a 65 year old Italian man from central eastern Italy. After completing schooling at 17 years of age, he emigrated to Australia with his family. At the time of his stroke he was Managing Director of a highly successful smallgoods manufacturing and distributing business. The family was an integral part of business and home life. Although he had a good understanding of English prior to his stroke, Mr. S. had always been anxious about his English being understood, retaining a strong Italian accent and making some grammatical errors. At his factory, most employees were Italian and so it was common for Italian to be spoken there. His four children were well-educated and well-travelled with a high standard of both languages. He maintained close contact with his brother in Italy with whom he shared an interest in vineyards and wine production. Written communication in Italian was therefore important.

The impact of the stroke was significant on Mr. S. and his family. He adopted a "sick role" within the family, such that early contact with health professionals met with strong resistance. He was also highly distressed at first with what he saw as loss of memory when the word finding difficulty of his aphasia caused him to be unable to recall the names of his family and friends. Having been head of the family unit and now highly conscious of his difficulties, Mr. S. showed particular distress at exposing errors to his wife. He preferred to sit back and let others anticipate his needs rather than ask and have his requests not be understood.

Following his stroke, Mr. S. presented with moderate receptive and expressive aphasia in both Italian and English. He reported that Italian was easier for him and, as that had been the language spoken at home and at work, an early recommendation was made that the family speak to him in Italian. He responded much better in both languages when there were additional clues of gesture and voice inflection. To plan appropriate management, the speech-language pathologist, an English speaker with only a basic knowledge of Italian, was faced with the need to determine the extent of impairment in an aphasic whose language experience had predominantly been in Italian. Comprehensive assessment of his primary language was deemed essential. A decision was made to use an interpreter rather than involve his wife as Mrs. S., with her emotional involvement and natural helpfulness, tended to influence the response of her husband. Furthermore Mr. S. was concerned about exposing his failure to his wife.

Assessment using translated Italian test material indicated that, as had been the case before his stroke, Italian was superior to English in speaking, understanding, reading, and writing and that there was no confusion between the two languages. A decision was then made to give parallel therapy in both Italian and English. One daughter, a teacher, was happy to take on this role with her father, given guidelines from the English-speaking therapist. With his daughter having the status of a teacher, Mr. S. was able to maintain his dignity within his family. Concurrent therapy in English was given for a number of reasons. Firstly, as both languages seemed to have been affected to similar degrees, relative to his pre-stroke skills, it could be anticipated that recovery might also be parallel. Secondly, this allowed the speech-language pathologist to provide a sound therapy model in English for the daughter to then adapt in Italian. Furthermore, while Mr. S. expressed a preference to speak Italian, the family expressed the need for rehabilitation in the language of his wider social and business environment.

As with Mrs. W., Mr. S.'s preferred and most successful language was his first language. However, unlike Mrs. W., Mr. S. was confronted with an English-speaking therapist with limited knowledge of Italian whose task was to determine the nature of his impairment and plan therapy accordingly. Questions were immediately raised about the language of assessment, complicated in the case of Italian speakers by the diversity of dialects spoken in Italy and the need to identify an appropriate interpreter. The role of the family in both the assessment and management phases was an important consideration due to both the bias introduced by helpful family members and the embarrassment experienced by Mr. S. in his altered role in the family. The need to train interpreters in the complexity of the assessment process was apparent. Adaptation of assessment tools where, at that time, only English resources were available was also necessary. As writing was an important means of communication, adequate resource materials were also necessary to tap reading and writing skills in Italian.

Language preference and degree of usage needed to be considered as vital components of the motivation and recovery processes. As English was less frequently spoken, even in the work environment, it was not considered appropriate as the sole language of intervention, nor was it considered appropriate to treat only in Italian.

Mr. S.'s emotional state and cultural beliefs needed to be considered at all stages. Acknowledging general health care beliefs, the "sick role", and changing family dynamics were integral to successful management. The potential involvement of family versus trained bilingual workers in ongoing management was also highlighted. This raises many issues related to the economics and practicalities of training and supporting other personnel. Where family were willing to be involved in management, the impact of this on Mr. S. needed to be balanced with therapy objectives. In some instances, it is neither possible nor preferable for all therapy to be carried out by family members.

Case Study 3

Mr. A. is a 43 year old Muslim Macedonian man who was identified, incidentally, as having had a stroke by an anaesthetist who was taking a pre-operative history. He was subsequently referred to a speech-language pathologist for confirmation of language problems. His English was described as poor by the referring doctor who suggested an "Italian interpreter." Both Mr. A. and his wife spoke very little English while their adult son and daughter were fluent in both Macedonian and English. Mr. A. was an invalid pensioner who had a circle of friends who spoke Macedonian or closely related languages.

During his initial contact with the speech-language pathologist, Mr. A. reluctantly explained that he was no longer able to read in his native language although writing in Macedonian was still possible. English literacy had never been established beyond a basic level. He further explained that he had kept his problems from his family, not wishing to alarm his wife or appear foolish in front of younger school-aged son. When receiving letters from his family in Macedonia, a regular and important event in his life, he would pretend to have lost his glasses and ask his eldest son to read the letter for him.

Given the speech-language pathologist's total lack of familiarity with the Macedonian language and Mr. A.'s limited comprehension and use of English, it was considered essential to have a trained interpreter to accurately and objectively assess the nature of his problem. Certain attitudes needed to be taken into account when selecting an interpreter. Due to the relatively small Macedonian community (the Macedonian population in the city of Perth was at that stage approximately 14,000), confidentiality was a concern for Mr. A., creating wariness and suspicion of the assessment process. He also expressed a reticence to have a female interpreter. This attitude was further reflected in his preference to confide in male members of the family and in his perception of males being the decision makers.

Given Mr. A.'s problems with reading, a major task of the interpreter was to assist in the assessment of his literacy skills. When asked to write a letter to his parents in Macedonian, the interpreter was able to verify that this was grammatically correct with occasional spelling errors and some minor evidence of interference from English. Reading, however, was impossible. He was limited to reading single letters and only able to identify a word if it was sounded out. All other reading tasks were too difficult. Mr. A. was diagnosed, at this time, as having "alexia without agraphia" or "impaired reading with intact writing."

The role of the interpreter included communicating the outcome of assessment to Mr. A.'s highly anxious extended family, in particular, his wife. As the identification of such reading problems was strongly indicative of Mr. A. having had a stroke, the need for further neurological investigation had to be communicated along with discussion with the doctor regarding implications for Mr. A.'s future health. Involvement in therapy, however, raised different issues. As therapy was complex and required regular and frequent sessions, it was considered essential to enlist the help of family. Mr. A.'s daughter-in-law who spoke fluent English and Macedonian agreed, with Mr. A's consent, to carry out the treatment program. While Macedonian was the primary language in therapy, functional reading for general life-skills was also targeted in English after Mr. A. expressed frustration at not being able to carry out routine reading tasks in English.

Mr. A.'s case highlights the cultural and linguistic barriers facing the bilingual aphasic when two cultures meet. Given Mr. A.'s reluctance to let others know of his problem and the difficulties an English-speaking professional would have in identifying the exact nature of his reading problems, the value of an interpreter was paramount in both identifying the problem and planning intervention. A monolingual English approach to assessment would certainly have led to misdiagnosis as Mr. A.'s literacy levels in English were not sufficient to highlight the problem. Identifying his reading difficulties then enabled the further diagnosis of a probable stroke to be confirmed, leading to management decisions beyond Mr. A.'s language problems. The essential role of the interpreter in communicating with family, both in relaying accurate assessment information and in reducing anxiety and isolation, was also highlighted. A monolingual professional is often powerless to assist the family in this vital area.

Choice of interpreter was also a key component in this man's management. Mr. A.'s concerns over confidentiality within the small cultural group in the community and his preference to work with males both needed to be respected in the selection process. Delicate issues relating to political sensitivity of the interpreter also arose with Mr. A.. This situation is not uncommon when political and social conflicts are occurring in the aphasic's country of origin. All issues discussed earlier, in the case of Mr. S., relating to the training of interpreters in the assessment process were also pertinent to Mr. A.'s management. This was particularly important in relation to the intricacies of the reading and writing systems.

The language of choice for intervention was clearly Macedonian given Mr. A.'s relative competence in the two languages and the fact that he frequently received letters from his family in Macedonia. Competency was greater for both spoken and written language in his earlier acquired language. Interestingly, some therapy was carried out in English for day to day survival skills at Mr. A.'s request.

An understanding here of the strong cultural influence behind Mr. A.'s denial of his illness due to its perceived sign of failure was necessary. This allowed an appreciation of Mr. A.'s reasons for hiding his difficulties from his family and facilitated a successful plan of treatment that was sensitive to this attitude. Furthermore, the initial reference to Mr. A. being "Italian" highlighted the potential confusion in language and cultural stereotyping and the need for expert assistance in selecting interpreters.

ISSUES CONFRONTING THE BILINGUAL APHASIC

The histories described above are by no means isolated ones. In clinics throughout Australia, aphasics from a multiplicity of cultural and linguistic backgrounds come into contact with the health care system and must face a whole set of different issues that relate both directly and indirectly to their bilingualism.

The Australian population is a conglomerate of people whose origins span one hundred and twenty countries. There are approximately eighty different immigrant languages currently spoken throughout the country[21]. In addition, one hundred and fifty Aboriginal languages are spoken although Lo Bianco[14] reports that only approximately fifty of these remain viable. Less has been documented on the contact of Aboriginal language speakers with the health system as these languages tend to be restricted geographically to the center and the north of the country, away from the main centers of population. While English is the only language spoken by 83% of Australians, between 15% and 20% of the Australian population daily use a language other than English[14]. A study of the aphasic population in Australia in 1985 found that a similar proportion of bi and/or multilingual aphasics was presenting to speech pathology clinics[24]. Using a survey that included 1,730 patients from large acute hospitals in most capital cities in Australia, the incidence of bi and/or multilingualism in aphasics was found to be 15.8%, extending as high as 22% in some clinics.

Mrs. W., Mr. S., and Mr. A. are therefore representative of a significant proportion of the aphasic population in Australia. They highlight the multiplicity of issues that confront bilingual aphasics and impact on their lives and their recovery. These can be broadly divided into language, culture, support personnel, and resource availability issues.

Each is elaborated below.

Language Issues

As is clear from all the above cases, effective management of bilingual aphasics from the viewpoint of speech-language pathologists requires a clear understanding of a range of issues, many of these directly related to the language difficulties experienced by the aphasic. Not only must the speech-language pathologist be aware of the impact of neurological trauma on language but also of the need to seek assistance in gaining some insight into the linguistic systems and competencies of the bilingual. This will directly influence assessment procedures and practices and the overall management of the aphasic and the family.

Grosjean[10] presents a holistic view of bilingualism that stresses the integrated nature of the two languages in an individual. Grosjean states:

"The bilingual is NOT the sum of two complete or incomplete monolinguals; rather, he or she has a unique and specific linguistic configuration. The coexistence and constant interaction of the two languages in the bilingual has produced a different but complete linguistic entity"(p. 6).

In the case of the bilingual aphasic, this unique picture must be considered when attempting to determine the extent of breakdown in the different languages. The importance of this, for example, in selecting and administering monolingual aphasic test batteries cannot be overstated. Grosjean elaborates on the limitations of assessment batteries designed for monolingual aphasics when used with bilingual aphasics. By their very nature, most standardized tests do not consider the different needs and social functions of different languages nor the complexity of the interaction occuring between them.

Paradis[18] also addresses the attempts in the literature to seek discrete differences between monolinguals and bilinguals as a way of understanding the bilinguals' language system. He further reports on the inability to make too many generalizations among bilingual subgroups, stressing the disparity among such groups even when such attributes as sex, degree of proficiency, age, and manner of acquisition are taken into careful consideration.

Any interested person who embarks on a scrutiny of the literature in this area over the years will notice the strong interest in investigating the nature of language recovery in the bilingual aphasic. The varied patterns in the recovery of the respective languages are well documented by Paradis[16] whose work has been a welcome contribution to the debate on how the different languages respond to both trauma and recovery. The debate has stretched the continuum from Ribot[20] who proposed that the earliest learned language, the native language, recovered first, to Pitre[19] who suggested that it was the most recently used language that showed initial recovery. This has evolved, through Paradis, into an awareness that the question of recovery is far more complex and varied than earlier theories had indicated. The implication for speech-language pathologists working with bilingual aphasics is that no general rules exist for clinicians to follow when targeting language for intervention. The pursuit of rules to predict which language would be the best facilitator for language recovery would seem to be too variable to be productive. The need to constantly monitor the relative impairment and improvement of the different languages, along with the interaction between the two, is clearly demonstrated in the case of Mrs. W.. In order to promote optimum language recovery, no predetermined pattern of language return was anticipated or used to guide practice. Instead sensitivity to individual preference and recovery patterns dictated management decisions.

Policies that aim to assist the speech-language pathologist in making decisions on language choice in both assessment and therapy are, however, being increasingly formulated. Such recommendations are not driven by research into patterns of language recovery but by a sensitivity to cultural and familial preference. The *American Speech-Language-Hearing Association*[1] recommend that assessment of speech and language impairment, where English is not proficient, should take place in the client's primary language. The *College of Speech Therapists*, United Kingdom, in "*Good practice for Speech Therapists working with clients from linguistic minority communities*"[6], recommend using both or all

> ". . . the languages which clients use or are exposed to in their daily lives to differentially diagnose the language impairment and to counsel and remediate"(p. 1).

The College further suggests

> ". . . the decision about the language(s) of therapy must be influenced by the nature of the client's linguistic repertoire, which may be bilingual, or non-English, or have the sociolinguistic expectation of being bilingual"(p. 10).

These recommendations not only reflect the **preference** of the aphasic but also the **rights** of the aphasic in an increasingly multicultural society such as Australia. The *Australian Language and Literacy Policy*[4] promotes the rights of cultural identity, social justice, and economic efficiency whereby an individual's cultural and linguistic heritage should be respected, developed, and used, regardless of background.

The direct implication rests with the speech-language pathologist having a clear appreciation of the nature of bilingualism and approaching the bilingual aphasic as a complex and unique individual for whom assessment and management need to be tailor-made. This is not a new concept for any speech-language pathologist. Within the aphasia literature on the monolingual aphasic over the last decade, there has been an increasing number of studies addressing models of language processing and production[5,7,8,13,22]. These have demanded that the clinician look more closely at understanding the underlying cognitive and linguistic deficits found in aphasia and then manage accordingly. The investigation of aphasia in the bilingual is not exempt from this pursuit. What is raised, however, in the event of bilingualism and aphasia is an additional set of variables that do potentially impact on language breakdown. Paradis[16] identifies some of these variables as including the individual's age at which each language was acquired, the modalities and sociological context of acquisition of each language, the context and modalities of usage, the degree of proficiency, as well as the affective value attached to each language. It is through looking at these factors that speech-language pathologists will find some of the answers to their questions regarding appropriate management of the bilingual aphasic.

Cultural Issues

An increasing body of literature highlighting the cultural implications of language loss has also been gathering momentum over recent years. Much of this stresses the need for health professionals to be sensitive to the cultural mix that is likely to arise within the individual and, where possible, to become familiar with the practices and beliefs of the cultures with which they are working. Anderson[2] succinctly summarizes this view when she states:

> "To achieve cultural sensitivity and a respect for different cultures, it is necessary to desire to learn more about different peoples, languages and cultures as well as about one's own culture. Such broader knowledge will probably bring with it the realisation that there are many more similarities than differences across cultures, but that these small differences are important and greatly affect clinical interactions"(p. 9).

The importance of a sound knowledge base is equally stabilizing for the professional who can often feel very uncomfortable working with new cultures. *The College of Speech Therapists*[6] reports that:

> "Many speech therapists working with this client group feel their clinical competence seriously challenged by the linguistic and cultural differences which confront them"(p. 1).

An increased awareness and appreciation of such differences can therefore only work towards a more positive and productive outcome for both the professional and the aphasic.

The three aphasics described in this chapter exemplify the importance of taking a holistic view of the person, noting attitudes and preferences in relation to their past and present social milieu. As a recent widow, the link between Mrs. W.'s homesickness, her grieving, and the language of her stated and demonstrated choice could not be ignored. It was also very clear that her confused state, agitation, and depression reduced when hearing the more familiar Dutch language. Throughout Mrs. W.'s management, her success in therapy required sensitivity to this need. This was necessary both for her optimal language recovery and for personal reassurance. Later recommendations regarding integration back into her community supported the need to provide and maintain those links for cultural support that would be integral to her whole recovery.

Many of the features ascribed to southern European cultures are seen with Mr. S.. Maintenance of the "bella figura" was apparent in his resistance to wearing a splint for his arm and similar to his initial reluctance to attempt communication where he might make errors. The "physical self-concern syndrome," discussed by Minc[15], was manifested in Mr. S.'s constant need for reassurance of recovery and that he was receiving every possible available service. The role of allied health professionals was unfamiliar to him, hence the importance of family involvement in therapy was heightened. Further, there was conflict between rehabilitation objectives aimed at establishing independence and his socio-cultural expectations in the sick-role that needed to be acknowledged. Often a person will, as the "patient," see him or herself assuming a central role within the family and circle of friends with the expectation that family will forego normal activities and focus on his or her needs. The family's wish to then fulfill their participatory role in the recovery process also needs to be respected.

Mr. A. shared some of this naivety about the role of the allied health professional but in his case it was to accord the presumed all-knowing and powerful status of "doctor" to all people involved in his health care. With this attitude came a response of awe and, on occasions, mistrust. Once trust was established, however, he would remain steadfast in this and wary of involving others. This wariness, for example, was apparent in his use of an interpreter. While concerned that a female may be selected, he was more mindful of her role in his ever watchful and critical ethnic community as he perceived it. Reassurance of the impartiality and code of confidentiality of the interpreter was necessary. Furthermore, in a culture where the role of the male was predominantly that of provider and protector, Mr. A.'s unemployed status, coupled with his wife's limited English, needed to be handled with sensitivity.

There must therefore be a commitment by health professionals to understanding the effects not only of another language but also of a different cultural background. Furthermore the degree to which aphasics and their families have assimilated linguistically and culturally into their new environment will differ. Hence

> ". . . the key for speech-language pathologists in working effectively with ethnolinguistically different families is to do so with respect and an appreciation of each family's uniqueness"[2](p. 10).

All assessment and intervention practices should therefore be responsive to the bilingual aphasic's unique story.

Support Personnel

A significant issue raised in the above studies and particularly pertinent to the Australian context is the use of support personnel, i.e. interpreters and bilingual aides, to overcome the all too frequent language barrier. As discussed earlier, the aphasic is often confronted with a monolingual health environment, a situation that is becoming increasingly recognized as a dilemma for bilingual aphasics and their families and where solutions are being sought to overcome the difficulties faced by this group of people. In particular, there has been a realization that people other than speech-language pathologists need to be involved in the assessment of aphasics, both in gaining essential background information and in tapping linguistic abilities. To facilitate this, the training of support personnel has become a key strategy where other cultures are involved and usually involves an interpreter. While Mrs. W. was managed by a bilingual speech-language pathologist, interpreters were integral to the management of both Mr. S. and Mr. A.. The establishment of a collaborative relationship between professional and support personnel has usually formed the basis of productive practice with aphasics, extending beyond the training of interpreters to the training of health professionals in working closely and effectively with interpreters. *Australia's National Language and Literacy Policy*[4] strongly supports this philosophy, stating:

> "Interpreting and translating skills are fundamental to meeting communication needs of people of non-English-speaking backgrounds who do not speak English well, including many migrants, Aboriginals and the hearing and speech impaired. Interpreting and translat-

ing services ensure that lack of English is not a barrier to people's access to information and services . . ."(p. 98).

The cases discussed however highlight the complexity of this practice. The consideration of choice of interpreter, for example, raised in these cases has been documented in the literature. The importance of sensitive selection has been discussed by Emamy[9] who recommended, when working with Iranians in Australia, using

> ". . . male interpreters for males and female interpreters for females" and, ". . . if using a family member as an interpreter, only use someone from the immediate family, not extended family or friends"(p. 105).

The *College of Speech Therapists* supports the use of an independent interpreter in its recommendations[6]. Friends, relatives, and neighbors are discouraged due to the potential embarrassment to the aphasic along with the difficulties inherent in administration of testing procedures and relaying often complex, technical, and personal information to families. The systematic training and use of interpreters by speech-language pathologists in Australia is monitored through the Australian Association of Speech and Hearing National Advisory Committee on Multicultural Issues (ACMI). As part of their objectives, this group aims to ensure regular and ongoing training of interpreters and promote awareness and evaluation of policies pertaining to interpreters with communication impaired people[23].

While a host of issues are raised here in terms of the cultural demands and acceptability of interpreters for the bilingual individual, it is in almost no other area that the intricacies of language are more apparent. It is essential for the speech-language pathologist to obtain accurate information on the aphasic's linguistic status, a task that involves communicating the aims of assessment and management to other personnel with often limited formal language training. Responding to the need for highly informed interpreters, training courses have been developed. Speech-language pathologists working with bilingual aphasics are involved in formally educating interpreters within health services to assist in assessing and counselling bilingual aphasics and their families[24]. Such courses have recently been incorporated, in Australia, into those approved by the *National Accreditation Authority for Translators and Interpreters* (NAATI).

Hand in hand with education of interpreters is the need for education of health professionals and, in particular, speech-language pathologists. This group needs to be aware of efficient and appropriate utilization of these support personnel along with the importance, for example, of planning briefing and debriefing sessions for them. Knowledge of the subtleties of language and cultural differences are as important here as when working directly with the bilingual aphasic.

Resource Availability

The final area to be elaborated on here addresses the development of resources suitable for both assessing and treating the bilingual aphasic along with the need for their widespread availability.

The importance of the speech-language pathologist gaining sufficient historical information on the languages spoken by the bilingual aphasic has been alluded to earlier through Paradis' work. In obtaining a history of the bilingual aphasic's language behavior, Hilton & Kraetschmer[11] stressed that it is not enough to simply ask if the person "speaks another language," but that it is essential that a speech-language pathologist be aware of the person's premorbid linguistic competency in all modalities of language as well as such factors as relative preference, recency, and frequency of use for each language. While clinicians have often devised their own procedures to access this information, Paradis' *Bilingual Aphasia Test*[17] with its extensive case history format offers a comprehensive launching pad for this process. The *Bilingual Aphasia Test*, with translations in 40 languages, has a fifty-item questionnaire on the history of the aphasic's bilingualism. For each language, consideration is given to the environment in which the language was used, the age it was acquired, how often it was used, and the aphasic's own perception of competency in each language prior to the onset of aphasia. This information then serves as a guide to selecting appropriate subtests from the remainder of the test to tap language abilities.

Until recently, assessment tools that examined the complexity of language breakdown with the bilingual aphasic were limited. Speech-language pathologists either developed their own tools based on a scrutiny of the literature or adapted test batteries that were available in the primary language of their country which, in Australia, is English. This latter strategy, while it has probably been the most commonly used approach, has been fraught with problems. Many of these problems relate to the cultural history of the second language and, once again, to the cultural and linguistic differences between the two languages.

Cultural differences abound in the task of translating existing test material and relate to such areas as cultural and linguistic etiquette, geography, religion, and experience. Etiquette is seen most clearly in the forms of address that often arise in formal test translation. The assessor needs to remain sensitive to the different polite forms of address and the implications of age where older people often prefer the more formalized forms. Geographical considerations emerge with the translation of place names and climatic conditions. An example of this can be seen if the question from the *Western Aphasia Battery*[12], a Canadian test, "Does it snow in July?" were to be presented to a Taiwanese immigrant in Australia. Experience and general exposure to test items also present a potential source of error for the aphasic. Tasks where aphasics are asked to provide the names of objects may be influenced by total unfamiliarity with an object and also by the fact that objects may not have direct translations in different languages.

Linguistic differences present by far the most complex source of error in direct test translation. Literal or exact translations of test items are often highly inappropriate. Asking an aphasic from a non-English-speaking background to explain the direct translation of the idiom "It's raining like cats and dogs," another item from Kertesz' test battery, may indeed receive some interesting responses! Different grammatical features of the languages such as word order also become highly important and result in sentences not being translated word for word. With languages varying so greatly, it is highly likely that direct translation of the meaning will not keep the words in exactly the same order in the sentence or, if they are, the complexity of the sentence and task may well be changed.

Paradis' *Bilingual Aphasia Test* has filled a large void in this area and provided a useful starting point in the assessment of aphasics from bilingual backgrounds. The complexity of detail considered in each language to ensure that assessment results are comparable across languages is impressive. Care has been taken, for example, to ensure that people in the test pictures are dressed appropriately for their culture, and climate and background scenery depicts geographical and religious beliefs, as in the dome of a mosque in the background of a scene in the Farsi version.

Therapy resources remain perhaps the least developed and available set of resources for the bilingual aphasic population. While a difficult undertaking in any country where many different languages prevail, there is a need for speech-language pathologists to be working together with other bilingual speakers and developing this area. Adaptation of communication aids, where appropriate, along with the translation and adaptation of specific therapeutic material needs to occur. Furthermore, the development of such resources should assume a priority at levels higher than simply the individual speech pathology clinic with involvement in resource development occuring at many tiers. Tangible therapy aids are however only one aspect. The development of sound therapeutic principles for working with bilingual aphasics must be promoted at all levels of health care. Ranging from a high profile of multicultural issues in the training of professionals through to ongoing action in the health-care workplace, an increased awareness and knowledge of this area must be encouraged. The development of competencies for speech-language pathologists working with minority language populations by the *American Speech-Language-Hearing Association*[1] has been one contribution to this ongoing task. In addition, the establishment of multicultural community networks is of central importance to management. Management of this population cannot occur separate from its own cultural milieu and hence links between and across cultures need to fostered.

In summary, through exploring some of the issues facing the bilingual aphasic coming into contact with the health professional in a monolingual English-speaking environment, the need for an increased awareness of the additional complexities of a bilingual and bicultural background has been highlighted. For aphasics and their families, the language problems experienced in a culture other than their own may be increased tenfold as they interface with a culture less familiar with their language and how it may break down. From the viewpoint of the speech-language pathologist, effective intervention requires a clear understanding of the impact of neurological trauma on different languages, sound assessment procedures and practices, and the continued development of personal and therapeutic resources. Of additional and vital importance in carrying out this effective intervention is the need for a widespread appreciation of the cultural implications of working with a multicultural population.

FOCUS FOR THE FUTURE

While the *College of Speech Therapists*[6] proposes that bilingualism "... is an advantage and rarely the cause or exacerbating feature of any disability" (p. 1), it is indeed the case that factors extraneous to the actual linguistic deficit can significantly influence the diagnosis and course of the aphasia and severely restrict communicative success. Bilingualism is not a disadvantage in itself but a monolingual environment, if unsupportive, may not be optimal for the aphasic and family. For this reason, responsibility rests at a number of different levels to ensure that the optimum environment is created. A summary of some of these responsibilities and how they may be implemented are broadly outlined below.

The professional, with particular reference to the speech-language pathologist, has responsibilities at both a micro, or clinical level and a macro, or policy level. At a clinical and individual level, the professional should ensure a commitment to,

- maintain a sensitivity to the issues facing people from bi/ multicultural backgrounds that relate to their assimilation into their new environment as well as those relating to the cultural attitudes that arise in coming to terms with the aphasia and the health care system;

- develop a knowledge of the languages of the aphasics with whom they are working and the interplay between the language and the culture;
- work with interpreters to gain a comprehensive history of the bilingual aphasic to make informed and sensitive decisions on language of assessment, counselling, and therapy;
- assess the aphasic with a sound understanding of the nature of bilingualism and how this will influence the type of assessment and the choice of assessment material;
- plan management considering the aphasic's language needs, preferences, and environment and incorporate appropriate material and personnel;
- continue to develop human and material resources for bilingual assessment, counselling, and remediation; and,
- encourage and participate in research related to the management of bilingual and English-speaking aphasics.

On a macro level, the professional needs to have a broader agenda and have an input to policy development at government level. The *Australian National Policy on Languages*[14] states that,

> "no Australian resident ought to be denied access to medical and health assistance . . . because of language disabilities, or lack of adequate, or any, competence in English"(p. 8).

For speech-language pathologists to implement this in relation to the bilingual aphasic, the infrastructure needs to be created to support the principle of equality of service so that assessment and management can be offered in the language matched to the aphasic's needs. This would require lobbying from the profession to,

- increase the component on bilingualism and cultural variation in the training syllabi of all health professionals, especially speech-language pathologists;
- recruit more bilingual speech-language pathologists from linguistic minority groups;
- develop specialist posts for speech-language pathologists and bilingual co-workers;
- conduct in-service training for all health professionals on issues related to bi/multilingualism and bi/multiculturalism, in particular, speech-language pathologists and bilingual co-workers;

- establish the national accreditation level required for interpreters working with speech pathologists through contribution to courses;
- establish support networks for ongoing needs assessments and provision of resources;
- formulate policy statements for speech-language pathology services reflecting recognition of the needs of their clients in the linguistic minority communities;
- lobby for supportive holistic environments, particularly in such places as nursing homes for the elderly; and,
- advocate for the rights of bilingual aphasics and their careers.

Finally, while the professional and society must take stock and reflect on this sizeable population of aphasics presenting to clinics and in the community, the aphasic remains the key player. The spotlight must remain on the aphasic as a whole person with needs, rights, and reactions to the aphasia that has changed his or her life.

REFERENCES

1. American Speech-Language-Hearing Association (1985) *Clinical Management of Communicatively Handicapped Minority Language Populations.* ASHA: June 1985.
2. Anderson, N.B. (1991) Understanding cultural diversity. *American Journal of Speech Language Pathology*: Sept, 9–10.
3. *Australian Bureau of Statistics Census of Population and Housing* (1986) Canberra: Australian Government Publishing Company.
4. Department of Employment, Education and Training (1991) *Australia's Language: The Australian Language and Literacy Policy.* Canberra: Australian Government Publishing Company.
5. Caramazza, A. (1986) On drawing inferences about the structure of normal cognitive systems from the analysis of patterns of impaired performance: The case of single case studies. *Brain & Cognition,* **5,** 41–66.
6. College of Speech Therapists Specific Interest Group in Bilingualism (1990) *Good practice for Speech Therapists working with clients from linguistic minority communities: Guide-lines of the College of Speech Therapists.* London: College of Speech Therapists.
7. Coltheart, M., Sartori, G. & Job, R. (1987) *The Cognitive Neuropsychology of Language.* London: Lawrence Erlbaum Associates.
8. Ellis, A.W. & Young, A.W. (1988) *Human Cognitive Neuropsychology.* London: Lawrence Erlbaum Associates.
9. Emamy, M. (1989) The Iranians. **In** *Culture & Health Care.* Perth: Health Department of Western Australia.
10. Grosjean, F. (1989) Neurolinguistics, beware! The bilingual is not two monolinguals in one person. *Brain & Language,* **36,** 3–15.
11. Hilton, L. & Kraetschmer, K. (1983) International trends in aphasia rehabilitation. *Archives Phys Med Rehabilitation,* **64,** 462–467.

12. Kertesz, A. (1982) *The Western Aphasia Battery*. New York: Grune and Stratton.
13. Lesser, R. (1987) Cognitive Neuropsychological Influences on Aphasia Therapy. *Aphasiology*, **1**, 3, 189–200.
14. Lo Bianco, J. (1987) *National Policy on Languages*. Canberra: Australian Government Publishing Company.
15. Minc, S. (1963) Of new Australian patients, their medical lore, and major anxieties. *Medical Journal of Australia*, **1,** 19, 681–687.
16. Paradis, M. (1977) Bilingualism and Aphasia. **In** H. Whitaker and H. Whitaker (Eds) *Studies in Neurolinguistics*. New York: Academic Press.
17. Paradis, M. (1987) *The Assessment of Bilingual Aphasia*. New Jersey: Lawrence Erlbaum Associates Inc.
18. Paradis, M. (1990) Language lateralization in Bilinguals: Enough already! *Brain & Language,* **39,** 576–586.
19. Pitre, A. (1895) Etude sur l'aphasie chez les polyglottes. Revue de Médecine, **15,** 873–899. Translated **in** M. Paradis (ed) *Readings on Aphasia in Bilinguals and Polyglots*. Québec: Marcel Didier.
20. Ribot, T. (1882) *Diseases of Memory: An Essay in Positive Psychology*. London: Paul.
21. Senate Standing Committee on Education and the Arts (1984) *A National Language Policy. Parliamentary Paper No. 3/1985*. Canberra: Australian Government Publishing Service.
22. Seron, X. & Deloche, G. (1989) *Cognitive Approaches in Neuropsychological Rehabilitation*. London: Lawrence Erlbaum Associates.
23. Stacey, K. & Sjardin, H. (1991) AASH National Advisory Committee on Multicultural Issues (ACMI). Report given to the Multicultural Issues Forum at 1991 AASH Conference. *The Australian Communication Quarterly*, Summer Edition, 18.
24. Sjardin, H. & Whitworth, A. (1986) *Dysphasia in Double Dutch. Bilingualism — Its implications for aphasia assessment and intervention.* Workshop presented at Australian Association of Speech & Hearing, National Conference, Hobart, Tasmania.

CHAPTER 9

THE PERSON WITH APHASIA AND THE FAMILY

D. LABOUREL AND M.-M. MARTIN

INTRODUCTION

The family is the first group to which an individual belongs, and, in most cases, it is the primary reference group. As people pass through the various stages of life, the family represents the total or partial setting for privileged interaction. Yet individual variance in autonomy or creativity can lead to the tightening or loosening of family ties. When a man or woman faces a crisis in adulthood or adolescence, fundamental relationships may be called into question on all levels. The flow of time and the unfolding of events are interrupted and their course is altered. The extent of the disruption and change will lead persons with aphasia into various forms of relationships which can be considered with relation to opposition and complementariness.

The family, like a biological cell, is affected by internal and external relations. The nucleus is the couple and their children. Nearby is a second unit — the other relatives — that either covers the nucleus or exists independently.

Illness, in this case aphasia, spurs a tightening or a slackening of family bonds. The family's reactions are influenced by the pre-existing relationships as well as by their responses to the upheaval. The aim of this chapter is to examine the effects of aphasia on the interaction of family members with the person whose communication is impaired following a brain injury.

ALTERATIONS TO FAMILY RELATIONSHIPS OVER THE COURSE OF THE ILLNESS

Onset of the Illness

When aphasia occurs, invariably an unforeseen event, family life is temporarily frozen so that each member may attend to the urgency of the patient's survival. The health-care world is the singular preoccupation; for a time, life is subsequently reduced to a functional biological existence.

The hospital context thus takes on the role of the new family: The hospital itself is an omnipotent mother, with a horrifying regressive dimension. The father is represented by the physicians' medical knowledge. Time is suspended while a host of worries and hopes come to the surface. The family members can be said to be mere onlookers to a gigantic reorganization of basic facts, a genuine "sudden rebirth" or a tragic incomprehensible death. Everything that is said at this point, in reality or in fantasy, will have enduring effects on the main characters of this drama.

The Return Home

Once they leave the hospital or rehabilitation center, persons with aphasia distance themselves to some degree from vital concerns. From now on, everything occurs in one setting — the home — with changes to adapt to and old habits to rediscover.

Familiarity will gradually set in. The family attempts to find a common ground between two worlds — that of the person with the illness, and that of the healthy members. The role of each member will be compared, with a view to adapting the needs and interests of the patient to those of the family. The disability thus finds a place in the family (it may even take up all **the** space). There is an awareness of a changed environment. The absence of the person that was hospitalized is now filled by the presence of a stranger; at any rate, one stranger exists: the illness.

Defense mechanisms are put to the test as the individual, the couple, and the family undergo structural changes. A new equilibrium is sought on the basis of an illusion, or disillusionment.

Stabilization of Progress

Persons with aphasia gradually carve out a place in the family, the cell which surrounds them, while the other members get accustomed to the changes in their environment. After several long months, or even years, families learn to live with the effects of aphasia and drift towards realization of the limits of rehabilitation. Looking back upon the progress of persons with aphasia and their families that we have known, it seems that the family and the patient pass through identical stages. The patient determines the general direction of change, primarily through the various aspects of his/her personality, but also by the degree in which the other family members become involved with that person. The impact of the symptoms of aphasia is another influential factor.

The severity of the disability and the length of the rehabilitation period are major determinants of changes within the family. If the rehabilitation and dependency stage is brief, couples or families may not necessarily undergo significant transformation. The change in roles is slight, and the difference is not overly troublesome. Thus, before too long, the former social order is nearly reinstated.

Unfortunately, the same cannot be said for persons who experience severe, lasting disabilities. Below is a discussion of these persons' personal and family life.

A PERSON WITH APHASIA IN THE FAMILY

The person with aphasia is an intimidating presence in the family. He is ashamed of his deterioration compared with his former capacities; he is pitiful and solicits indulgence like a child or a person with a mental deficiency. The person with aphasia can perceive these attitudes and suffers as a victim of this fate. He may feel that the illness is a punishment: "Why did it happen to me?" What, in his past, in his former lifestyle, could justify this devastating blow?

The person's need to rationalize this event which upset his whole way of life may lead him to blame the *other* for remaining silent and allowing the illness to occur. That other person is guilty of neglect and abuse. Faced with this inexplicable fate, it is essential not to reveal any weakness.

Within their families, persons with aphasia are living behind a facade. Everyone is pretending that nothing has changed, yet the persons' actual presence is a painful role in the drama. They find themselves excluded from discussions and decisions. Many persons with aphasia have reported being *frightened,* a fear akin to stage fright — a dread of people.

The person with aphasia must get used to the fact that tasks which were formerly simple are now challenging. The old routine and habits are no longer valid. Telephone calls, interaction with salespeople and neighbors are all met with a sense of panic, speech is often blocked. Persons with aphasia have no confidence in their abilities; they anticipate failure. Therefore, they prefer to avoid this discomfort and they withdraw from social contact. By losing themselves in the family environment, they can fade into obscurity.

Relations within Couples

It is difficult to grasp what transpires within a couple when one of the spouses acquires aphasia. Often, the person most qualified to deal with the couple's difficulties is the speech pathologist, since this person is the specialist with whom the patient forges a significant (and often enduring) alliance. Here are a few basic features of this relationship.

- Changes occur over time. Therapists become increasingly familiar with the patient's situation and gradually become involved in the patient's progress. They are also witnesses to the spouse's acceptance or exclusion of and adaptation to the person with aphasia.
- According to the sex of the patient and therapist, transfer, identification, and projection responses can be observed and may influence the relationship. These reactions may also surface between the therapist and the patient's spouse.

The illness and aphasia represent a major crisis within the family; this leads to a reorganization of the fundamental relationships. The illness occupies a permanent place as a third party; sometimes an ally, sometimes an enemy. Initially, depending on the therapist and the context, the spouse may be described as overprotective, spoon-feeding, encouraging, or active (even hyperactive). He or she may even wish to direct the language exercises, to play a leading role in the person's recovery.

Generally, speech pathologists are adept at identifying and limiting this initial zeal which, because it consumes too much energy, quickly leads to exhaustion and deception. The spouse can assist in rehabilitation on another level, one which relates to elements of private life. These include everyday verbal and non-verbal exchanges and situations experienced in their natural settings. It is impractical to recreate artificial communication situations between the spouses; exercises, homework, and programs should be handled by the patients themselves. The extraordinary effect of this dissociation between automatic and voluntary behavior is most evident in everyday life.

Shyness and guilt often inhibit the spouse from acting naturally with the person with communicative and other disabilities. Implicit attention, and listening to persons with aphasia, however, can encourage them, increase their self esteem, and enable them to maximize their residual capacities.

Anguish, fatigue, and depression drain the *spouse* of availability, patience, and inventiveness. Many couples get aggravated and exhausted by the endless riddles. Daily activities often cause dissatisfaction and isolation, leading each spouse to retreat into a separate parallel existence. Healthy spouses immerse themselves in outside activities, take charge and assume all responsibility, while the spouses with aphasia confine themselves to the home, thus retreating from dreaded social contact.

Since these persons did not actually choose the status imposed by the illness, they turn possessive and become demanding towards the healthy spouse who lost nothing and enjoys everything that they now lack, but which was formerly theirs. In couples where one of the spouses has aphasia, the bonds (or lack of unity) become more intensified; the situation before the illness is heightened. The result is highly revealing (similar to developing solution that causes images to appear on photographic paper). From then on, the essential characteristics of the relationship between the two partners will become keenly visible.

When Martha, the household authority, decision-maker, and manager, acquired Broca's aphasia, she became tyrannical, demanding, and possessive of her weak, pathetic husband who never dared to motivate her.

Stella's experience was comparable, yet her reactions were kinder and gentler since she was previously of a more pleasant disposition.

The actual circumstances that these couples faced led them to extreme reactions, despite the counselling and the warnings offered to them. Feeling trapped, the husbands felt and stated that they could not act otherwise. To others, their total self-denial seemed, at times, inconceivable, even indecent. These women lost their autonomy, and were unable to take care of themselves. Because their husbands were too domineering and oversolicitous, these patients were unable to satisfy their intimate and most basic needs.

In other cases, men with aphasia and severe disabilities often find themselves being spoon-fed by their wives. Here again, overprotection and excessive assistance can impede rehabilitation and recovery. In this situation, the therapist represents a refreshing external presence who, for a fleeting moment, conveys a different message. What more can the professional do? Action cannot be forced upon the patient. In such cases, therapists can contribute through their presence, attentiveness, and exemplary behavior.

Naturally, in couples who are fifty years or older, the scope of the readjustments will be highly limited. The years of sharing will have cemented many attitudes. In addition, the common experiences will also increase the likelihood of the couple's acceptance of any disabilities and will allow them to make proper choices regarding compensatory techniques. The harmony resulting from decades as a couple and the powerful bonds forged by hardship and joy are extremely meaningful for some couples, and should encourage them to maintain their mutual respect and energy to stay together despite the occurrence of aphasia.

In younger couples, it is not only the present but also the future which is found to be fundamentally altered. They are often forced to abandon their dreams, hopes, and goals in life; mourning is all the more difficult when what is lost never really had the opportunity to fully materialize.

The rupture and loss exist not only for the person with aphasia and for the couple, but also for the healthy spouse, whose hopes are also dashed. Healthy spouses find that they are the only ones able to preserve the couple's identity. They must set aside all the hopes that they invested in their mate. This requires analytical skills and flexibility that are far from universal traits.

The damage induced by the illness, the castration brought on by aphasia, elicits defense mechanisms in each spouse which enable them to cope with the crisis. These reactions also vary between couples. More specifically, the dependency arising from the disability will be dealt with differently by each partner.

In Peter's case, it was the independence of each spouse that was reinforced. His communication was impaired by his limited verbal abilities (severe dysarthria) and comprehension difficulties arising from verbal deafness. Each spouse worked at a demanding job. Peter's residual ability to communicate through writing allowed him to return to work. They each went about their own business, sometimes meeting for a shared meal with the children. Each partner went on separate vacations. Peter could not tolerate noise and the children's activities. Instead he withdrew, reading or listening to music. His wife was highly committed to her job, and ensured that the household preserved a "normal" appearance.

Sally acquired aphasia and hemiplegia soon after the birth of her daughter. In addition to relentlessly pursuing a rehabilitation program, she devoted considerable energy to raising her child. Her dominant role in the couple allowed her to retain her status in the household. Aggressive by nature, she did not succumb to regression or dependency. She consistently maintained the image of an elegant and active woman, always finding things to do at home, and remaining attentive to her husband.

Christopher has had aphasia and hemiplegia for ten years. He was forced to quit his job as a salesman. After he spent several years rehabilitating, his wife found him a place where he can keep himself busy and a gain a sense of usefulness. His good nature and congenial character endear him to the children, who see him every day during lunch break. The couple continues to see friends and plan vacations. They share a reciprocal respect which they preserved despite the disabilities induced by the illness.

The bonds maintained by this couple helped them overcome their problems. The strain, however, can be unbearable for other couples. Some wives or husbands can no longer see aspects of themselves in their partners who have undergone drastic changes. Although they may feel guilty, they prefer to distance themselves and live apart.

Adam's wife found herself in this situation. After several years of helping her husband recover basic communication skills, she realized that she could not remain a wife to this person who was no longer the man she used to love. Because of the deep respect she had for him as a human being, she could not bear to remain with him out of pity or pretence. She finally mustered the courage to leave, granting him the promise of an amicable relationship over the telephone.

Beatrice was severely disturbed by her aphasia and hemiplegia. She could not accept her disabilities, and became bitter and aggressive. Although she was initially quite attractive, her self-image soured once she acquired aphasia. She gained weight. Her husband evidently gave up, discouraged by Beatrice's negative and self-destructive behavior. He could no longer rationalize sharing his life with a woman who was averse to any planning or hopes for the future.

Defense mechanisms, denial of the disability, depressive phases, and crisis resolution all emerge at varying stages and degrees for different people.

The speech pathologist, apparently not excluded from all these events, is often a key figure in the couple's life. He or she becomes a third party, and may be ascribed various roles.

- ***Ally*** of the person with aphasia. In principle, the therapist understands the problems of persons with aphasia, and possesses various tools to help them. Sometimes the therapist will be privileged enough to better decode the person's rudimentary communication. He or she will subsequently reap a reward: The first stammering and attempts at communication; a situation which may incur the jealousy of the spouse.

  This apparent secret alliance can have positive repercussions. It is a sign of progress which will be demonstrated and elucidated to the spouse, who should be encouraged to participate in the process. The therapist will then distance him or herself personally from the relationship with the person with aphasia so that their interaction can serve as a model and a frame of reference. The speech pathologist needs the patient's trust. It is generally easily granted, while that of the spouse is often harder to earn.

- An ***invader*** of an individual or a couple's private life, due to the severe trauma of the loss of language. This loss significantly narrows the range of communication, and, curiously enough, focuses it on "the self," easily exposed without reserve or inhibition.

  This aspect of aphasia has grave consequences. The idea "Actually, you know all about me" is extremely disturbing for the person with aphasia. It rouses the spouse's suspicions, and, naturally, must be taken into account by the speech pathologist. Therefore moderation, discretion, and confidentiality should all figure prominently in therapy sessions.

- ***Master of thoughts and deeds.*** The speech pathologist proposes one task or another, and suggests reading materials and activities not only to the person with aphasia but also to the spouse.

  Tact and respect can ensure that the therapist will be heeded, and that the advice will be carried out. The role described above must be handled prudently, given the danger of dependency inherent in this relationship. In fact, the language disability quickly and easily leads to submission and the loss of initiative. The role of the speech pathologist is to assist patients in recovering their will and autonomy at the same time as they are assisted in regaining their language abilities. Therapists also instill in patients a more positive self-image and enhanced personal dignity.

In addition, the speech pathologist represents:

- a ***witness*** to the conjugal relationships that are, to some degree, strained, tense, or even disrupted. The person with aphasia feels victimized, stricken a second time. He perceives an injustice in that he cannot confidently engage in human interaction, especially on an emotional level (partly because of personality changes, but also due to the neurological deficit which hampers control over moods). The feeling of deterioration increases, exacerbated by the idealized memory of his former condition. "I feel like everyone is looking at me." Why is the person with aphasia under this impression? Perhaps this question should be turned around so that we can ponder whether he himself is capable of *observing* others, particularly his spouse.

Parent — Child Relationships

Persons with aphasia experience a loss of authority since they are less able to issue orders, directions, and explanations. This powerlessness, sometimes mistakenly viewed as indifference and aloofness, causes persons with aphasia to withdraw emotionally and distance themselves. They may periodically display violent reactions — pressure valves for their internal tension. The illness also puts many events into perspective, sometimes life itself. Persons with aphasia may become fatalistic and passively endure the onslaught of worries and questions. Can anything else happen to them that would be even more damaging?

Child-rearing becomes the exclusive domain of the spouse, supplemented by meaningful looks from the present but powerless person with aphasia. Therapy sessions often offer a glimpse into the person's helplessness in complex family interactions.

The father's role is particularly threatened. Because of the illness, men with aphasia tend to become housebound, and sometimes willingly engage in traditionally female activities such as domestic chores; others strongly oppose household duties. A new equilibrium is eventually reached with unfamiliar dimensions and roles.

Young children may suffer considerably due to their inability to comprehend the reasons for the parent's communication impairment. Fortunately, children are gifted with the ability to communicate extralinguistically. In many cases, children quite naturally become the allies of the person who is no longer the same as the other family members.

For example, Kimberly learned to talk thanks to her mother's stammering, gleefully repeating her paraphasic utterances. Little by little she became her mother's main confidante, guessing or whispering what she attempted to communicate, as well as expressing her opinions to people in the outside world.

The father of young children who acquires aphasia develops a closer relationship with his offspring, who benefit from his increased presence in the home. He is frequently an enthusiastic audience for their speeches and tales. The child benefits from a friendly ear, and, essentially, compensates for the conversation that is lacking in the father.

In this situation of trust and natural exchange, the parent with a language deficit may recover linguistic elements through the dissociation between automatic and voluntary speech. He can boldly express his ideas, and can speak to and teach the child because he is not afraid of criticism of his poor language abilities. Conversations about school, and reciprocal correction add to the interaction and liven the dialogue in which each speaker will find (or rediscover) new information. Note that this secret alliance may occur only on occasions when parent and child are spending quality time together.

Parents with aphasia often have difficulties explaining the rationale behind certain decisions, voicing opinions, and answering the child's questions. When they manage to express opposition, they often do so with excessive emotion: aggressive reactions that border on violence. In contrast, other persons may turn to stone and withdraw, unable to express themselves. Anger or seeming indifference are two manifestations which disturb the person with aphasia, causing a particularly painful frustration.

Peter's eyes always brim over when he discusses his son. He writes "my boy." The son's displays of instability and insolence are met with considerable indulgence. What do the child's repeated provocations mean to him?

Sally, with severe aphasia, was devastated over not being able to teach her child to talk. She was distressed that her daughter was distorting words the way she did, and did not speak like other children. She was extremely frustrated at not being able to glance through picture books with her child, to discuss the illustrations and invent stories around them.

Maria, mother of a four-year-old girl, found great solace in her daughter, who did not attend school until the age of six. The child was thus a companion to her mother and facilitated contact with the outside world. Unfortunately, although reassuring and comforting to the mother with aphasia, this particular relationship ultimately burdened the child with emotional, social, and school-related difficulties.

Adolescents react towards parents with aphasia with the strong and forceful impulses which characterize this stage of life. They experience episodes of worrying and uncertainty which may rekindle problems of identification. They are disturbed at not being able to find a stable role model either in the disabled parent, or in the other parent, who is often unavailable and is trapped into a role through no choice of their own.

The disabled parent is seldom mentioned in the company of friends. Their existence is hushed up, their *words* are nonexistent. Pretence is the rule so that feelings will not be hurt. Crucial subjects are not discussed.

When he talks about his father, Justin laments: "With him, I can't discuss work, girls, or the future, so I just give up."

Adolescent girls sometimes become protective and maternal, leading to indulgence and a setting aside of essential problems. They may also play key roles as helpers to the person with aphasia. Clarice delayed going to boarding school; she intended to abandon her studies to remain with her mother, who had aphasia. Stephanie wanted to become a speech pathologist, having had natural experience communicating with persons with speech impairments.

Many factors influence a child's reactions and adaptation to a parent's aphasia. Below are the most determinant elements:

- the age of the child at the time of the traumatic event, and the identification problems which characterize each period;
- the quality of the relationship between the parents, and the ensuing family atmosphere.

Relationships with Relatives

Depending on the speaker, the word "family" may refer to one's family of origin, parents, siblings, aunts and uncles, and perhaps even the spouse's family — the *in-laws* — with whom affectionate bonds and familiarity will vary according to past experience, affinities, and circumstances. Members of the *extended* family may provide support to the *sick unit* or, on the contrary, may be perceived as intruders and a threat to the person's fragile equilibrium.

The illness causes people to ignore conventional behavior; affinities and bonds will now arise spontaneously. People who are unable to express themselves or make themselves understood become dependent upon others to communicate their needs and to voice their ideas and emotions. Sometimes a brother-in-law or an aunt will be most adept at decoding the speech of the person with aphasia, who can no longer communicate like everyone else. Note that someone who is less of a blood relation to the person by his or her availability and previous knowledge of the patient, can be in a better position to understand the person's reactions or intentions. Below is a discussion, based on examples of a few families, which should shed light on the different types of relationships that may come into play.

After he acquired aphasia, Bill developed a special relationship with his unmarried sister. Each day she comes to work with him; she attends to his paperwork and helps the children with their homework. Aphasia creates a need for reparations; it gave Bill the opportunity to express his dependence upon and also his power over his sister. She, in turn, found in her brother's home a sense of worth and responsibility that was lacking in her solitary existence.

Louis M. is often alone during the daytime. His wife works outside the home and his children attend trade school. Mrs. M. decided to move when her husband returned from the rehabilitation center. She found a house near her parents, who live on a farm in a nearby suburb. Louis M. visits the farm daily, where he assists his father-in-law by doing odd jobs or caring for the livestock.

Peter is no longer mobile. He cannot read and his speech is barely comprehensible. His mother-in-law lives in the same neighborhood and often visits for part of the day to keep him company when his wife is at work or out shopping. His father-in-law, too, spends time with him on occasion. They both enjoy living at a slow pace and watching television.

Karen, 20, is another unhappy person with aphasia. She was forced to leave school, and devotes much energy to rehabilitation. From time to time she treats herself to a break in her routine — a visit to her grandmother's home, where she had spent many a school holiday. There she is indulged as a child once again. With her grandmother, who eagerly accepts her, Karen can temporarily forget her constant struggle to overcome her word-finding problems.

Availability, warmth, and encouragement are not the only possible qualities of relationships between persons with aphasia and their loved ones. Indeed, aggression, misunderstanding, and rejection from one or both sides may occasionally surface. Rivalry may be expressed freely when one of the people involved can no longer defend himself.

Take Diane's family, for example. Diane's speech is unclear, she cannot find words, she tires easily, and cannot plan her activities and errands. She, who was the heart of the household, who gave of herself to all the other members, today is dependent and indecisive. The slightest annoyance makes her edgy, and she can no longer bear solitude. Her siblings by no means provide the support she requires. They continue to harass her over the division of the father's estate, they snub her when she calls on impulse, and they do not understand the couple's problems. They view her merely as an aggravating and embarrassing woman who does not know what she wants.

Mary J. does not live in the calmest environment imaginable. This dynamic and athletic woman cannot tolerate her hemiplegia and her language deficit, and, as a result, has become domineering and violent. She vents her frustrations on her sister, who cares for her with the help of Mr. J. Since Mary is unable to control her aggressive outbursts, the hapless sister has become the scapegoat for all her hostility.

These cases demonstrate that the *extended* family may complement the family nucleus. Persons with aphasia may turn to these relatives for availability and understanding. They need someone to share their slowed lifestyle, someone to whom they are neither spouse nor parent. Yet these relatives are close enough to them that they will likely understand the persons with aphasia despite their reduced or unintelligible speech. The greater capacity to listen may be linked to the fact that the disability affects the extended family members to a lesser degree, and does not pose a threat to their relationships with the persons with aphasia. Likewise, they have less need for defense mechanisms, and can accept reactions which are intolerable for the person's spouse and children. Persons with aphasia, in their family of origin and among their in-laws, may be perceived as children; this will enhance acceptance of regression and impotence. A not uncommon observation attests to this situation: Some women with aphasia revert to using their maiden names in their signatures.

RELATIONSHIPS OUTSIDE OF THE FAMILY UNIT

The Person with Aphasia along with the Family

Persons with aphasia often have difficulty maintaining the social relationships that they enjoyed before the illness. In general, it is the spouse who presses the person with aphasia to meet people who are significant in his or her life, such as in-laws, friends, or colleagues.

The behavior of persons with aphasia in society often mirrors their behavior at home. They may either withdraw or demand full attention, which is either a reflection of their personality before the illness or an entirely different reaction.

Bob has extreme difficulty articulating; his wife usually speaks on his behalf. Most often he will let her proceed, resigning himself to wrinkling his brow or shrugging his shoulders. Occasionally he will convey outright disapproval with a growl. When his wife is engaged in conversation, he will perform endless gestures to attract her attention and to convey his impatience.

As for Bill, he became quite talkative since he acquired aphasia. When he visits family or friends with his wife, he monopolizes the conversation and attracts everyone's attention. People are then forced to decode his agrammatical speech. His presence, which is always strongly felt by others, conveys the impression of a dynamic and attentive individual. He commands the attention of everyone he meets; his aphasia is never met with indifference. His wife can only go along or leave him be.

Marvin gets easily annoyed when he is unable to say what he wants, or when he utters erroneous words. He no longer appreciates the presence of others in his home to the same extent; he is annoyed that he cannot assert himself with others. Without warning, he will retreat to his workshop in the garage.

In the outside world, with people who are *unaware*, aphasia amplifies disagreements to a greater extent. Often, the person with aphasia wants to be recognized as a disabled person, while the spouse attempts to camouflage the disability and strives to maintain the appearance of a normal couple at all costs.

Diane and her husband are victims of this phenomenon. The spouse, neither sociable nor talkative by nature, cannot fathom that his wife needs contact and communication with other people, regardless of the sometimes disjointed quality of her speech. Diane has slowed down, and is highly sensitive to any attention bestowed upon her. For her, the changes in life brought about by aphasia represent an opportunity to live differently, and she seeks authentic rather than mundane relationships. Her husband, ill at ease when it comes to personal problems, flees from precisely the interaction that his wife seeks.

Distancing and aggression are, of course, not the sole reactions within a couple when one partner is stricken with aphasia. Take Eric R., for example. Four years after the onset of aphasia, he and his wife evolved towards a state of respect and mutual support that allowed both to express themselves at their own pace, according to their own interests. After difficult periods of misunderstanding, rebellion, and depression, calm was restored to the household and a new equilibrium was reached.

Mrs. R. lets her husband ramble on in confusion, even once she has guessed his meaning. As a result, he is not as possessive and as demanding as before, and she is no longer required to constantly attend to him. They visit friends and entertain in the home. When they travel, she explains to others why her husband has problems speaking. Naturally, this harmonious state, despite the aphasia, is linked to the quality of the relationship that the couple enjoyed before the illness.

In the outside world, it is the couple that is perceived as aphasic. Aphasia, accepted and compensated for by *the spouse*, is not an obstacle to interaction with people who view the illness-related difficulties only from afar. In contrast, in cases where one of the partners constructs defense mechanisms such as denial, rejection, and overprotection, encounters with family members or friends will be painful and quite strained. As a result, people who do not know how to respond to this considerable friction will tend to marginalize the couple.

The Person with Aphasia outside of the Family

The house, protective but also isolating, is not always the place where the person with aphasia feels most comfortable. Dependent and powerless, unable to speak, persons with aphasia who must face their loss around loved ones often enjoy solitary excursions, and a rather autonomous existence.

Once he acquired aphasia, Richard lost the ability to pursue his profession, and found himself unemployed and house-bound. He soon suffered from cabin fever. Now he pays regular visits to a group of acquaintances in the neighborhood who bowl together. With them, he is accepted and appreciated. While playing, he can voice his disapproval and rejoice in a fine performance. With his bowling partners he is an ordinary man.

Peter, too, likes to venture out alone. He prefers solitary vacations, especially ones involving travel. Abroad he no longer has aphasia, he is simply someone who does not master the language of his travel destination.

Although persons with aphasia avoid certain situations because they cannot experience them as before, in other contexts they may wish to preserve the power or the knowledge previously acquired.

For most men, driving is an essential activity; sitting at the wheel of one's car is highly symbolic. The car allows them to regain power, and in this active albeit automatic role, they can become independent and strong.

Participation in other types of leisure activity is also quickly renewed. For some, fishing is an excellent form of escapism since it requires little or no speech! Games such as chess and checkers are characterized by ritualized encounters where prolonged speech is not necessary.

Joel can no longer maintain his position as manager of a firm. He has a loss of sensitivity in his right hand, yet he insists upon paying daily visits to his billiard team, where he strives to outdo his long-time rivals.

Persons with aphasia but not hemiplegia may give the impression that they are able-bodied. As soon as something unexpected or unusual occurs, however, they may quickly panic. Because they cannot verbally explain their fright, they may present maladaptive behavior. Some persons with aphasia may flee, while others may exhibit uncontrollable outbursts of violence.

Recovering their autonomy and braving the outside world once again is an essential need for most persons with aphasia. They may feel a bit more like themselves when they are not among family members, since they are no longer reminded of their disabilities and limited by the family's expectations. Some persons with aphasia, when responsible for themselves, with no one to remind them that some things are not done in society, use their disability to its greatest advantage.

Matthew, for example, exaggerates his comprehension difficulty and purposefully conveys the impression of having a mental deficiency. At the Social Security office, he is allowed to go to the head of the line so that he will not attract too much attention. The disability, an embarrassment for the companion of the person with aphasia, is sometimes brought to the forefront by the person himself, who then successfully commits himself to the companion's absolute care. Rick's case is such an example. He was constantly watched over by his wife, who feared that he would make a careless mistake. One day he staged an impromptu escape to visit a female friend in nearby Paris. Unfortunately, no one was home at the address where the taxi dropped him off. His funds depleted, Rick feigned illness on a public bench. He was then taken to the hospital. His wife was contacted and eventually arrived to pick him up.

The person's autonomy and external relationships are highly contingent on his or her personality. Other influential factors include the immediate family's encouragement or deterrence of outings by the person with aphasia, who no longer enjoys the same status.

Outside of his normal setting, the person with aphasia may feel freer, or on the contrary, even more threatened. He will come across new situations which he will handle according to his abilities. In these contexts he is capable of manifesting other aspects of his personality, and his limitations no longer make him pine for his former self. Some persons, however, find it overly difficult explaining their evident deficits, and fear interaction in highly uncertain situations. They therefore limit their outings to a restricted area where they are already recognized as persons with aphasia.

Persons with Aphasia and their Friends

The relationship between persons with aphasia and their friends is often a painful topic. At the same time as the persons with aphasia condemn their friends' detachment, they themselves provoke the friends' retreat and strain amicable ties. This distancing is more or less desired by the persons with aphasia, who do not wish to be in an inferior position or to experience problems. Their reserve is sometimes perceived as an aloof invulnerability.

Gradually, the gulf of mutual incomprehension deepens, one which the person with severe disabilities may no longer be able to bridge. Contact is generally strained. Persons with aphasia feel that these changes affect the magnitude of their own personality and those of others. "Now I am small, and others are big," is how one person explained his isolation. How do persons with aphasia cope with this regression and devaluation? Do they refuse to compare themselves with others, and rely only on themselves?

The shock of facing aphasia in a familiar and respected individual may spark unexpected, intense, strange, and even selfish reactions in friends. Statements such as: "It's beyond me, I can't stand to see my friend like that," "What would we talk about?" and "Everyone has his cross to bear, it's really unfortunate" are commonly heard among the person's circle of friends. Soon enough, the friends resign themselves, unable to counter this tragic fate — to immediately or effectively soothe the suffering. They feel that they cannot bear to be around the person with aphasia. They cannot be helpful if there is so little that they can offer. Those who attempt to analyze their retreat from the person with aphasia confess to harboring feelings of confusion. Adam's friends, faced with his severe communication difficulties, no longer consider him to be the same person. They cannot tell what he is thinking. They are no longer certain of their role in his life.

They report that they fear the extent of the changes, and they feel guilty towards the person who is so diminished. What has become of their common past? What future can they now hope to share? Part of them was consumed by the illness that transformed their friend into someone who is not capable of verbal communication.

The true friend, whose devotion is revealed during the painful stages, offers regular and discrete support, listens attentively, and provides dynamic help to stimulate the person's interests. That person may propose activities and organize outings. This friend has no need to find him or herself in the other person, and can tolerate differences. Often the person will have undergone a traumatic experience which taught him or her to put events in perspective, along with the value of an unconditional presence.

The initiation of new relationships is generally limited, since the person with aphasia has often become suspicious and vulnerable. People who cannot appreciate the extent of the disability — the constant foe of the person with aphasia — may shy away. In fact, many people hide behind their aphasia and use it as a facade. This is particularly true of young adults and adolescents who have not had the opportunity to forge enduring relationships. They rarely and only with great difficulty succeed in overcoming the feeling that they are misunderstood by others. They do not wish to feel undervalued, nor diminished by harsh critics. Victims of fate, they distance themselves from their peers, whom they tend to idealize. They are easily disappointed and dare only to risk small portion of themselves in partial relationships.

Fear of the unknown and difficulties in acknowledging differences naturally create problems in the initiation of sexual relationships. Very few young single persons with aphasia enter into satisfying sexual relationships and raise families.

Cynthia, a dynamic and enterprising woman, is surrounded by friends. She is demanding a lot from the people she meets; she wants to form a large unified family. The ties that she tenaciously and zealously creates offer her support and reassurance. Some people perceive them, however, as chains that Cynthia has used to bind them. This emotional interaction is affected by varying perceptions of the relationship; freedom may be experienced in contrasting ways. Karen cannot always find someone to go out with during the evening or on the weekend. Aphasia, which occurred early in her studies, alienated her from her friends. She and her friends drifted apart; some moved in with boyfriends, others entered the workforce. They no longer have common lifestyles due to their contrasting activities. Karen has become quite cynical and demanding. She often spends time with older people because they have more time or indulgence to offer her.

Peter had many friends before his illness. His house was often filled with revellers listening to music or playing pool. Since he acquired aphasia, his house is considerably quieter and emptier. He spends long periods alone, occupied with books and music. Because they represent his past, few friends are *allowed* to penetrate his personal territory. Furthermore, he can no longer easily participate in their current lifestyle.

THE PERSON WITH APHASIA WHO LIVES ALONE

The Person with Aphasia without a Family

Persons with aphasia can live alone, in total autonomy, as long as their physical condition permits (if they do not have hemiplegia). They are thus mobile and can manage the household. They are able to shop in the neighborhood by patronizing familiar vendors, and by serving themselves in stores. They make payments by check if they can write numbers and do not mind waiting in line. Most often they will offer the cashier a bill of large denomination, and will pocket the change, which they assume to be correct (some persons with aphasia are unable to calculate). Bank cards also represent much appreciated tools for these persons who are uneasy about handling money.

Transactions in administrative offices can be facilitated if people present their aphasia identification cards which outline their disabilities. This card is an important psychological support that gives persons with aphasia the courage to tackle unfamiliar activities and face a world that they consider unbending and uncaring. The card also encourages listeners to be more attentive to the persons' requests, despite the awkwardness of their verbal expression.

Resigning oneself to solitude is a gradual process. Isolation is a distinct likelihood for those who naturally tended towards solitude. Some persons with aphasia live a silent existence, withdrawn into themselves; their inner richness allows them to devote themselves to their private lives.

These persons need to develop a full intellectual life. They spend much time with records, books, and collections. Some write, while others paint. Satisfaction is derived from energy used to recover former talents. To these activities, they devote their time, their strength, and their lives. They feel an urgent need to rehabilitate, displaying willingness, energy, and perseverance.

Over time, they experience a growing need to communicate to others what they underwent during this difficult struggle. Solitary persons with aphasia often mask the communication gap by committing their story to the pages of a journal, an activity which proves highly enriching for the author. It is a form of retraining of written language, and is a particularly effective means for grouping together all the elements of the person's personality as he solves the puzzle of life. By examining themselves at different stages and seeking links with the past, persons with aphasia may recover a zest for life.

Eric, who acquired jargon aphasia and agraphia, today divides his time between essential domestic activities, despite the boredom and fatigue that they induce, and literary creation, i.e. the demanding occupation of an author. The outline of his current novel is based on his personal life. It testifies to the bitterness and desperation of someone who was *bled dry* by aphasia. The purpose of his work is a search for appeasement, self justification, and intellectual challenge. Eric's inner richness and willful personality enable him to live in total retreat from the world. He is preoccupied with the past, and searches for his lost persona.

Bill, who acquired aphasia during adolescence, still experiences a considerable impairment of written language. He works in a protected environment at an activity that suits his abilities but fails to match his former objectives. His passion for painting assures him an active social life. His image as an artist has become a disguise for his disability and his solitary lifestyle. He maintains somewhat superficial contact with other people and, discouraged by past failures, is disinclined to take many risks. In general, everyone who is severely affected by aphasia experiences a psychic and emotional fragility that hinders the exploration of possible avenues.

Other Reference Groups

Although the family may provide refuge and a sense of belonging, it is not the sole reference group for most patients. For many able-bodied people as well as persons with aphasia, the workplace is extremely significant and may constitute a second family, especially in certain professional contexts. The regularity and duration of contact in the workplace can create strong relationships. Certain persons with aphasia may belong to sports teams, leisure groups, or other associations. Membership in a social group reinforces an individual's self image. Very often, this image differs from the role the person held within the family. For example, the structure of the work team, or the independence of unsupervised work may give people the opportunity to express personality traits that may not have become apparent in the family environment. For certain persons with aphasia, these satellite groups are the only contexts where the persons receive recognition and where they can reap enjoyment and moral support.

In the professional milieu, the continuity of a friendship will depend on the type of responsibility involved in the person's job, and the familiarity which existed before the illness. Sometimes persons with aphasia can no longer tolerate the loss of their former abilities. In other cases, colleagues become suspicious and misunderstand the changes in the person with aphasia. Relationships with colleagues may subsequently be disrupted, a severe blow for the person with aphasia, who may no longer be able to return to his former workplace. In other cases, support and generosity preclude discrimination, and relations remain intact. The persons are kept informed of all work-related events which concern them; they are even invited to occasional staff meetings.

Sports is often a traumatic topic since, quite often, persons with hemiplegia and aphasia, as well as other persons with aphasia, can no longer engage in their favorite pastime. Perhaps the person can still participate in a supportive or organizational capacity, letting others profit from his skills and availability. Leisure clubs may provide the opportunity for the person to spend time in a regularly scheduled activity; these groups offer warmth and much-needed distraction as well. Depending on the activities, the other participants may be more or less aware of the disability. For example, it is not necessary to speak well in order to appreciate stamp collection. Playing bridge, however, may become nearly impossible because most persons with aphasia find it difficult to follow the bidding. Other preferred activities include chess, checkers, and even scrabble, as well as certain card games.

Aphasia, since it brings about such drastic changes in lifestyle, may represent an opportunity to explore new activities and settings. For example, Lily, who sometimes suffers from loneliness, signed up for a walking club, and she participates in weekend outings where she has the opportunity to meet new people. The ability to develop a new identity is essential because comparison with the former self is precluded. Lily currently lives fully in the present, and does not mope over her loss.

Reactions to the disability and its place in one's new lifestyle vary widely according to the person's personality. Some people seek situations or contact that minimize the disability (at any rate, one where the disability is not prominent). Others, on the contrary, seem to have a constant need to refer to it, and wish to be viewed as nothing other than persons with aphasia.

Today, in most large cities, there are associations for persons with aphasia where the disability is the common factor among the members.

Persons of all ages, from all social and cultural backgrounds, spouses, siblings, parents and friends, all gather to exchange information, compare experiences as well as making the most of the residual capacities of persons with aphasia. These associations provide settings for the recognition and defense of the person's disabilities. They are also warm and friendly environments for people who find themselves without resources.

CHAPTER 10

THE FAMILY OF THE PERSON WITH APHASIA

R. BOISCLAIR-PAPILLON

INTRODUCTION

Of all known illnesses, aphasia is probably the one which affects the family most directly. Because of the abrupt, unexpected, and often permanent damage to communication, the entire network of family interaction is disturbed. Buck[4] justifiably qualified aphasia "the family illness."

The family is often considered to be a stable and balanced system where each member plays a predetermined role which complements that of the other members. Satir[16] views the family as a homeostatic entity, analogous to the homeostatic physiological state where each unit is dependent on every other unit. This mutual dependence implies that any change in one unit will consequently alter every other unit. Likewise, aphasia, which affects one member, will cause a disturbance in the equilibrium of the family and will bring about anxiety. This, in turn, leads to behavioral alterations in every other family member. Just as the person with aphasia influences the rest of the family, the family, also, influences this person's behavior, even the rehabilitation process.

This chapter will concentrate on the family's point of view. Without any doubt, the family of the person with aphasia also reacts to the illness and undergoes behavioral and attitudinal changes. Whether such reactions are extreme or moderate, supportive or destructive, they invariably stem from a disruption of the equilibrium. The direct link between family behavior and the recovery of the person with aphasia has been repeatedly demonstrated by authors such as Wepman[21], Buck[4], and Malone et al.[13]. The family plays a key role throughout the course of the illness: From the initial suspension of communication to eventual rehabilitation and recovery. The family's effectiveness can be enhanced by support from the therapeutic milieu.

Below we will examine the main reactions and changes commonly observed in families of persons with aphasia. We will also outline the role of the family in rehabilitation, as well as the necessary measures to enable families to best fulfill this role.

THE IMPACT OF APHASIA ON THE FAMILY

The sudden loss of the ability to communicate affects all aspects of the lives of the persons and their family. The therapist who has regular contact with the patient will observe the effects and subsequent reactions brought on by this disability. The emotional, relational, and social problems which plague the family, especially the spouse, have long been described in American studies[1,6,10,11,12]. We shall review the main disruptions below, along with commonly seen reactions and attitudes.

Changing Roles

Changes in familial roles and the difficulties that arise adjusting to new roles constitute a serious problem for families of persons with aphasia. In most cases, the spouse is suddenly faced with responsibilities and duties that formerly belonged to the partner. The healthy spouse not only becomes the sole bread-winner, but also must raise the children and attend to the management and upkeep of the house. Furthermore, the spouse with aphasia often requires particular care and attention. In cases where the person with aphasia was the sole source of income for the family, the disruption is even more drastic. Some spouses have reported feeling *crushed* by the multitude of responsibilities that were formerly shared.

Reactions to the role reversals are variable. Some people panic when faced with the magnitude of the tasks at hand, others discover previously untapped potential, and find the new roles satisfying, even rewarding. Once the person with aphasia returns home from the hospital, the couple may find it difficult to reallocate responsibility.

Given the evolution of the couple and the family in the past 20 years, clinicians have observed that reactions to role changes are less pronounced than before. In households where both spouses work, or where the couples habitually share financial, familial, and domestic responsibilities, the impact of the shift in roles is considerably less severe. Despite the magnitude of the task before them, the couple views the increased responsibilities as less overwhelming. Modern spouses are used to sharing tasks; to them it is only fair that the partner, even with aphasia, still occupy a place in the family dynamics and assume responsibilities compatible with the language deficit. In this scenario, there is a greater likelihood of achieving a new equilibrium.

Guilt

Many spouses feel guilty about the illness. Even today, the loss of the ability to speak is often viewed as a curse or divine retribution for past behavior. Others link the stroke to a stressful event, an argument, or to overwork in the days prior to the attack. Some spouses blame themselves for their inability to foresee the stroke and even accuse themselves of negligence, for not preventing it. The feelings of guilt usually linger, even once the person with aphasia returns home. In such situations, spouses may feel that they are not doing everything possible to attend to the needs of the person with aphasia.

Unrealistic Attitudes

Many spouses and loved ones manifest unrealistic attitudes about the patient's future. As reflected in studies by Malone[(12)], and Kinsella and Duffy[(10)], spouses of persons with aphasia tend to believe that improvement will take place, and that the person will eventually recover the ability to speak.

This hope intensifies when the person with aphasia begins treatment at a neurological rehabilitation center. Most spouses are convinced that the difficulties will dissipate over time, and that the person will resume former activities within a year, or two at most. Some insist upon more rehabilitation, even after therapy has been terminated.

Overprotection

Feelings of guilt often go hand in hand with overprotection. The majority of the spouses (81%) surveyed by Kinsella and Duffy[10] claim that they make every effort to avoid situations which may be stressful for the person with aphasia. Others admit that they themselves perform tasks that the person is quite capable of executing. They closely supervise the person's sleep, intake of medicine and food, and movement inside and outside the house. Public transport is forbidden, as are unaccompanied outings and the use of electric appliances. The person with aphasia is never left unattended in the home. Moreover, the spouses worry about the slightest problem or discomfort. A commonly-heard spouse's complaint: "I can't sleep, his slightest movement wakes me up!"

As a result, persons with aphasia become increasingly dependent and demanding on their spouses. For many spouses, the realization that it is they who induced this dependency often comes too late.

In many cases, overprotection disguises feelings of rejection. The rejection is not overtly expressed, but it is implicit in statements such as: "I consider my partner more of a child than a spouse."

Marital Relations

The loss of the ability to speak has a particular effect on the relationship between spouses. Couples experience problems with interpersonal communication, loss of feelings of togetherness, as well as a decrease in sexual satisfaction. Spouses find it difficult to discuss both everyday and special events. They are no longer able to communicate subtly their feelings and impressions. Each spouse will tend to be more reserved towards the other and friction soon escalates. Kinsella and Duffy[10] report that 83% of these couples abandoned sexual activity. All the spouses of persons with aphasia studied by Linebaugh and Young-Charles[11] claim to have undergone alterations in their marital relations.

Social Activities and Recreation

Social activities and recreation decrease in importance for all couples where one of the members has aphasia. A large proportion of couples complain of the social estrangement imposed by aphasia. Contact with workmates gradually dwindles, as does participation in social and church groups, and school associations, all of which may be fruitless, even impossible, for persons with aphasia. Group leisure activities are also suspended. Spouses of persons with aphasia, drowning in a multitude of tasks, have little time to devote to external contact. The couple rarely entertains or visits friends. Many people admit that they avoid discussing the spouse's disability with their friends; they also tire of constantly repeating the same explanations to each new listener. Little by little, former colleagues of the person with aphasia, friends of the family, and acquaintances all get shut out. Only the immediate family and perhaps one or two friends remain in the picture.

Each spouse and family member feels the repercussions of this disruption, and will respond to a different extent until a new equilibrium is reached. The nature of the adjustment is influenced by an array of variables such as the type and severity of aphasia, the physical autonomy of the person with aphasia, and his or her former personality as well as that of the spouse. Another influential factor is the spouse's involvement in the rehabilitation process.

THE ROLE OF THE FAMILY IN RETRAINING AND REHABILITATION

There are few clinicians who have never, over the course of their careers, observed a friend or relative of a person with aphasia who speaks rapidly to that person, incessantly interrupts, or even speaks in his place. Such attitudes are known to hamper the recovery of language skills. In contrast, attentive verbal behavior by the spouse or other family members can stimulate and even accelerate recovery.

Speech pathologists recognize that the general attitudes and verbal behavior within the family influence the effects of therapy. Williams and Freer[22] claim that patients without family support have a greater tendency towards physical and emotional deterioration; they also seem to benefit less from therapy.

How can loved ones, particularly the spouse, foster the re-emergence of adequate communication? Instead of simply being an observer, the spouse must participate in the treatment program and become an active member of the therapy team. Below we will examine the spouse's role during and after the person's period of hospitalization.

Source of Information

When persons with aphasia are admitted to a hospital or rehabilitation center, they may often feel isolated and unable to supply the information requested by personnel. Shortly after admission, the clinician consults the patient's family as to the person's linguistic behavior. Relatives can describe the person's language skills, verbal mannerisms, and particular interests. The role of language in the patient's life, the characteristics of his or her oral or written expression, and the presence of a pre-existing language defect are all areas to be explored.

The family, through observations of its own, is also able to provide insight into the person's communication problem. Spouses' appraisals are often useful since they can assess the past and indicate the patient's needs. What seems abnormal to the doctor may be totally acceptable to the family, and vice versa. Much depends on the environment and the patient's background, i.e. the social and medical history.

Webster and Newhoff[19] noted that it is preferable for the doctor to meet with family members as early as possible, since family members represent the *best historians* of the patient's condition and the events immediately following the stroke. In fact, the family is better able to preserve the image of functional behavior with its positive and negative elements.

Support and Stimulation

The progress of the person with aphasia is dependent on the preservation of social contact and the positive and encouraging attitudes of family members. Hospitalized, confined to an unfamiliar setting, and surrounded by strangers with whom they can communicate only poorly or not at all, persons with aphasia consider their spouse and children to be the only remaining link with reality. With their family, they can be understood without having to speak. It is only they who can interpret a gesture, a facial expression, or a posture, and communicate the meaning to others. Concurrently, they keep the person with aphasia informed of social, familial, and professional developments, immunizing him or her against isolation from the outside world.

The family contributes to the recovery of communication by supporting the persons with aphasia in their daily efforts to improve their communication. In certain cases, they can help the persons do things that they would be unable to do independently. It is essential that the family accept the changes and encourage the patient to persevere with therapy.

Regular presence of family members, coupled with close collaboration with the health-care team, can create a positive and stimulating atmosphere. Persons with aphasia strongly need such a support in order to sustain their motivation during the long months of treatment.

The family is in a much better position to provide support and stimulation for the person with aphasia once they are informed of the nature of the problem. Negative attitudes are usually seen in families who underestimate the communication disturbances, or who attribute the person's behavior to memory lapses, or to other cognitive defects.

Associate Therapist

Alongside the family's traditional supportive role lies a more specific one — that of associate therapist. The first authors to grant the spouse an active role in the recovery of language were Wepman[21], Rolnick and Hoops[15], and Helmick, Watamori, and Palmer[9].

The spouse, when informed of the objectives of treatment and of the therapeutic method, proves to be a key partner in the generalization and stabilization of relearned language skills. He or she loyally accompanies the person with aphasia throughout the stages of retraining, and supplements the therapist's task by helping with exercises that are prescribed outside of therapy. The spouse can also invent, in the course of daily verbal interaction, situations that will encourage the person to use the elements of language that were the object of therapy. The person with aphasia should also be encouraged to apply the techniques or strategies suggested by the therapist such as: delay word description, sound association, gestures, and mental imagery. Moreover, the spouse should be given tips on how to increase oral comprehension and expression in the person with aphasia, for example, by speaking slowly, giving the person ample time to talk, and refraining from interruption. The use of these facilitation techniques stimulates the emergence of functional language, and allows the patient to consolidate the skills learned in therapy. Florance[8] suggests that the spouse who becomes an associate therapist not only increases the effectiveness of therapy, but also diminishes the retraining period. Additionally, the spouse promotes the process of generalization and assists in assuring the permanence of progress.

Social Integration

During the first three or four months of hospitalization, the family is preoccupied by the immediate medical needs of the patient: physical well-being, morale, and physical and linguistic rehabilitation. Then comes the time when the person with aphasia is ready to reintegrate into the family unit. It is then that stress, as well as the physical, cognitive, and linguistic deficits, becomes fully apparent.

By adopting a supportive stance, the family can be of considerable assistance to the person with aphasia, who must adapt to changes in lifestyle and in family dynamics upon his return home. Gains achieved in therapy will be upheld and advanced only if the family encourages the person to use the functional language acquired. The family is also responsible for easing reintegration by promoting recreational activities, friendships, and other social contacts.

Certain attitudes may induce in the person with aphasia, a state of powerlessness which may eventually lead to depression. According to Malone et al.[13], families who persistently overprotect persons with aphasia, out of the desire to shelter them from embarrassment, actually contribute to their social isolation, which steadily worsens. Acceptance of aphasia, accompanied by open-mindedness, promotes social adaptation and a more satisfying use of functional language. Webster[20] described how the spouse's change of attitude and perception of the language deficit sparked the emergence of functional communication as well as changes in social behavior, despite the persistence of severe aphasia.

THE INTEGRATION OF THE FAMILY IN THE REHABILITATION PROCESS

Most centers that specialize in neurological rehabilitation now acknowledge the key role of the family in the recovery process. Some rehabilitation programs involve family therapy to allow the family to become significant and effective participants in the rehabilitation process. To accomplish this, families require adequate information, training, and psychological support.

Information

Most families have no prior experience with persons with aphasia, and are therefore faced with their first exposure to this disability. Confronted with a new reality, they are in need of adequate and reliable information on the nature of aphasia and its associated problems. Helmick et al.[9] reveal that spouses are poorly informed of the language disturbances associated with aphasia, and tend to minimize patients' comprehension difficulties. More recently, a study by Chwat and Gurland[5] measured the spouse's and children's knowledge of aphasia-related linguistic impairment. Few of the respondents were able to provide a complete definition of aphasia; none specified that comprehension difficulties were symptoms of the disability. The authors concluded that it is essential for the family to familiarize themselves with aphasia in order to better understand and accept the person with aphasia; such an acceptance will ultimately simplify their own lives. Many researchers concur on this issue.

Numerous pamphlets on aphasia and its consequences, such as the one published by a group of speech pathologists in Montreal[2], target families of persons with aphasia. Although the vocabulary is not necessarily that used by the general public, the documents generally contain pertinent information. At any rate, it is ultimately the duty of the speech pathologist to explain to the family the nature of aphasia, its neurological origin, its many manifestations, and the specific symptoms of each type of aphasia. Families will usually ask many questions about the prognosis, the factors influencing recovery, the duration of treatment, and the particular behavior of the person with aphasia in question. The therapist should in turn inform them of the objectives of treatment and the methodology being employed. The consent and collaboration of the family should always be founded on correct information.

Training

The primary target of therapy is, after all, the person with aphasia. In cases where the spouse or other family members are invited to participate in the rehabilitation process, they expect to receive training which will enable them to assist the person regain his language abilities.

Soon after the person's arrival at the rehabilitation center, the speech pathologist meets the family and discusses the initial observations. He or she describes the comprehension and expression disturbances that were revealed through the initial evaluation, as well as their manifestation in functional language. The speech pathologist will also encourage the family to adopt attitudes and behavior that will stimulate verbal communication. For example, family members will be advised to slow down their speech, avoid speaking too loudly, pause between words and sentences, and give the person with aphasia time to find words. In short, the therapist will relay the advice traditionally given to families in order to prompt communication.

At a later stage, the spouse or significant other will be asked to observe and participate in therapy. Therapists will then elucidate the patient's particular expressive and receptive disturbances. They will also relate strategies that are the most helpful for the person with aphasia. They will outline their methodology, specifying the aspects of language to be retrained. They will also discuss the techniques used to achieve the utterance or comprehension of words, or, as the case may be, the elimination of perseveration, echolalia, or other speech anomalies. These information sessions may be staggered over several appointments, the goal being to allow the spouse to pursue the work initiated by the therapist. The spouse will ultimately be able to effectively offer assistance on a daily basis by means of the exercises suggested by the therapist, and thus promote the emergence and generalization of functional language.

Spouses of persons with aphasia were found to modify only slightly their verbal and non-verbal communication, even when their partners had a blatant communication problem. Therefore, it is not surprising that interaction is often seen as frustrating and dissatisfying for both parties involved. In this case, it is preferable that the therapist encourage the spouse to embark upon a specialized training program.

Recent trends in aphasia rehabilitation stress the involvement of family members in the recovery of functional communication. Contrary to the traditional treatment model, many experiments have been performed in order to orient clinical treatment towards a pragmatic approach, thus favoring the integration of the spouse or loved one into the therapeutic process. This approach[7,14,19] is based on the analysis of communication in the context of conversation between persons with aphasia and their spouses, who are no longer mere onlookers but are instructed to interact verbally under the therapist's watchful eye. The object here is to modify specific behavior in the spouses' communication with the person with aphasia. An approach of this kind was successfully applied by Simmons, Kearns, and Potechin[17] in a program which focuses on training the spouse. The training targeted two types of behavior adopted by the spouse, i.e. interruption of the person with aphasia, and excessive use of convergent questions, which were judged to be interfering with communication.

Counselling

The occurrence of aphasia creates major upheavals within the family unit. In the critical early stages of the illness, the family, gripped by concern, devote themselves entirely to the patient's needs. Persistent communication disturbances tend to become increasingly evident to the family. At this stage, the desire to regain lost equilibrium and return to the former situation masks the severity of the deficit, and allows for a potential return to normality. The situation gradually becomes so overwhelming that the family is stricken by severe anxiety which causes them to withdraw further. They are apprehensive about the enormous responsibilities before them, and feel incapable of facing the disruption newly imposed by the illness. They are inclined to believe that they are powerless to alleviate the person's condition. Therefore, only the speech pathologist or the social worker can provide specialized assistance. Later, often with external support, the family reaches the stage at which they can cope with the situation, and play an active role in rehabilitation. At this stage they are more capable of evaluating the language problem, and can more realistically imagine the future with the person with aphasia.

Adequate information on the nature of aphasia and its consequences is essential from the early stages of the illness. This information is not, however, sufficient in itself; it must be accompanied by support from health-care personnel. Since speech pathologists are frequently in contact with the patients, they are well-placed to observe the emotions and concerns of both patients and their family. They should answer the family's questions as they arise. When therapists feel that there are problems that disturb the well-being of the patient and the family, they should not hesitate to recommend professional counsellors, such as social workers or psychologists. Such specialists can analyze the patients' behavior and help them clarify their ideas and emotions. Families often have a pressing need to discuss their emotions and reactions to the communication difficulties.

In Montreal, a solution was found in recent years to specifically meet the needs of these families: The aphasia support group. These groups keep families, particularly spouses, informed of the consequences of aphasia, and also offer assistance with difficult emotional, social, and familial adjustments. They tend to center around the following objectives:

- To provide information on aphasia, i.e. the pathology, the communication difficulties, as well as the associated cognitive and affective disorders.
- To give families the opportunity to share and discuss the problems linked to the person's return home, as well as daily life with a person with aphasia, and the changes induced by the illness.
- To provide a forum for the expression of feelings on the difficulties of life with a person with aphasia.
- To provide a setting for contact and moral support, thus diminishing the isolation experienced by families.

These groups are open to all family members, and participation is voluntary. They are primarily geared towards the close relatives of people who are currently undergoing therapy for aphasia. Yet spouses or children of people who acquired aphasia several years earlier can also benefit from these encounters. The groups are not structured; that is, items on the agenda are determined by the participants, or flow from their questions. The topics broached usually include: Communication problems, fears, the expression of negative feelings, difficulties adjusting, sexual anxiety, and changing roles.

It is generally admitted that such encounters, when combined with aphasia therapy, stimulate a rapid integration of the family into the rehabilitation process. Worries, anxieties, and problems are more rapidly identified by the therapists, and, as a result, dealt with before they become critical.

Another approach — that of family therapy — was introduced more recently. It concentrates specifically on the role of family interaction in the person's rehabilitation. Wahrborg[18] described it as an offshoot of psychotherapy, and distinguishes it from the support groups described above. The psychotherapeutic approach is simultaneously directed towards the person with aphasia and to family members, requiring their active participation. The composition of the group is preestablished and therapy sessions have a specific duration. Meetings are led by specialists who are experienced in psychotherapy and in neurology-related communication problems.

Family therapy stems from the notion that the aphasia-induced disruption to the family's communication system can often lead to psychological disorders and even depression. Therefore, it emphasizes relationships between the family members. Therapy consists of exposing the family and persons with aphasia to various situations, and encouraging participants to modify their negative behavior. The objective is to change the participants' attitudes in order to improve their general behavior, emotional reactions, social life, as well as their communicative abilities. Another goal is the alleviation of medical problems. This model, along with the implied therapeutic process, is inspired by psychotherapy techniques.

The family, as a unit, is thrown into disequilibrium when one of the members acquires aphasia. Before reaching a new balance where everyone finds a place, the family undergoes a metamorphosis and passes through a whirlwind of emotions and reactions. Persons with aphasia are influenced by the family's behavior. If the family is expected to play a positive role in the rehabilitation process, it is essential that family members not be left to fend for themselves. They can fulfill their essential role if the various therapists include them in the rehabilitation process.

REFERENCES

1. Biorn-Hansen, V.: Social and Emotional Aspect of Aphasia. *J.S.H.D.*, **22** (n°. 1): 53–59, 1957.
2. Boisclair-Papillon, R. & Coll.: *Vous connaissez un aphasique?*, Ministère des affaires sociales, Gouvernement du Québec, 1984.
3. Borenstein, P., S. Linell & P. Wahrborg: An Innovative Therapeutic Program for Aphasia Patients and their Relatives. *Scand J Rehabil Med,* **19:** 51–56, 1987.
4. Buck, M.: *Dysphasia: Professional Guidance for Family and Patient,* Prentice-Hall, Englewood Cliffs, 1968.
5. Chwat, S. & B.G. Gurland: Comparative Family Perspectives on Aphasia: Diagnostic, Treatment and Counseling Implications, **in** *Clinical Aphasiology Conference Proceeding,* BRK, Publishers, Brookshire, Minneapolis, 1981.
6. Davis, G.D.: *A Survey of Adult Aphasia,* Prentice-Hall, Englewood Cliffs, 1983.
7. Florance, L.C.: The Aphasic's Significant Other: Training and Counseling, **in** *Clinical Aphasiology Conference Proceeding,* BRK, Publishers, Brookshire, Minneapolis, 1979.
8. Florance, L.C.: Methods of Communication Analysis used in Family Interaction Therapy, **in** *Clinical Aphasiology Conference Proceeding,* BRK, Publishers, Brookshire, Minneapolis, 1981.
9. Helmick, J.W., T.S. Watamori & J.M. Palmer: Spouses Understanding of the Communication Disabilities of Aphasic Patients. *J.S.H.D.,* **41:** 238–243, 1976.
10. Kinsella, G.J. & F. Duffy: The Spouse of the Aphasic Patient, **in** *The Management of Aphasia.* Lebrun, Y. & R. Hoops (eds). Swets and Zeitlinger, Amsterdam, 1978.
11. Linebauch, C.W. & H.Y. Young-Charles: The Counseling needs of the Families of Aphasic Patients, **in** *Clinical Aphasiology Conference Proceeding,* BRK, Publishers, Brookshire, Minneapolis, 1978.
12. Malone, R.L.: Expressed attitudes of families of aphasics. *J.S.H.D.,* **34** (n°2): 146–151, 1969.
13. Malone, R.L., P.H. Ptacek & M.S. Malone: Attitudes Expressed by Families of Aphasics. *British Journal of Disorders of Communication,* **5** (n°2): 174–179, 1970.
14. Newhoff, M. & G.A. Davis: A Spouse Intervention Program: Planning, Implementation, and Problems of Evaluation, **in** *Clinical Aphasiology Conference Proceeding,* BRK, Publishers, Brookshire, Minneapolis, 1978.
15. Rolnick, M. & H.R. Hoops: Aphasia as seen by the Aphasic. *J.S.H.D.,* **34:** 48–53, 1969.

16. Satir, V.: *Conjoint Family Therapy,* Science and Behavior Books, Palo Alto, Ca, 1967.
17. Simmons, N.N., P.K. Kearns & G. Potechin: Treatment of Aphasia through Family Member Training, **in** *Clinical Aphasiology Conference Proceeding,* BRK, Publishers, Brookshire, Minneapolis, 1987.
18. Wahrborg, P. & P. Borenstein: Family Therapy in Families with an Aphasic Member. *Aphasiology,* **3** (n°1): 93–98, 1989.
19. Webster, E.J. & M. Newhoff: Intervention with Families of Communicatively Impaired Adults, **in** *Aging Communication Process and Disorders.* Beasly, D.S. & A. Davies (eds). Grune and Stratton, New York, 1981.
20. Webster, E.J.: A Spouse's Role in Rehabilitation, **in** *Case Studies in Aphasia Rehabilitation: For Clinicians by Clinicians,* Ed. R.C. Marshall, Austin, Texas, 1986.
21. Wepman, J.M.: *Recovery from Aphasia,* Ronals Press, New York, 1951.
22. Williams, S.E. & C.A. Freer: Aphasia: Its Effects on Marital Relationships. *Arch Phys Med Rehabil,* **67:** 250–252, 1986.

CHAPTER 11

THE PSYCHOSOCIAL ASPECTS OF APHASIA

M. HERRMANN,
H. JOHANNSEN-HORBACH,
AND C.-W. WALLESCH

INTRODUCTION

There is a multiple-way interaction between the various consequences of brain infarction and the patient's and his/her relative's psychosocial condition that precludes simple interpretations: Coping with chronic disability relies to a considerable extent upon psychosocial factors and psychosocial changes which are a result of chronic disease. This chapter will attempt to describe both psychosocial burdens and aspects of coping of aphasic patients and their families but will refrain from a detailed discussion of their various interactions.

Early empirical studies on the psychosocial consequences of cerebrovascular stroke tended to exclude aphasic patients because their communication impairment posed methodological problems. These "problems," however, highlight that aphasics are impaired in excess of the disability of other stroke patients[2] and that their burden should receive special consideration.

Figure 11–1 shows a simplified model of the consequences of cerebral lesion and various interactions between disease symptoms and psychosocial changes in aphasic patients.

I Aphasic symptoms are rarely the sole consequence of brain damage. Usually they are combined with various neurological and neuropsychological deficits that also influence psychosocial adaptation in different ways.

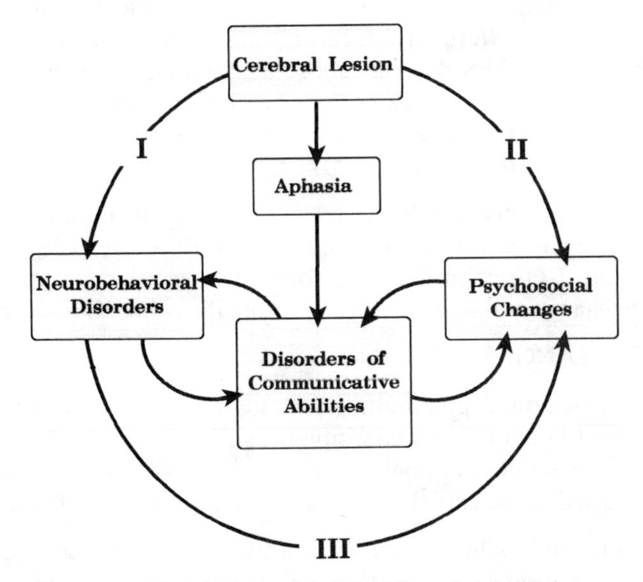

Model of Interactions between Disease Symptoms and Psychosocial Changes in Aphasic Patients.

Figure 11–1

II A vascular cerebral lesion affects the patient's and his/her family's psychosocial status abruptly. Compared with slowly developing chronic diseases there is no opportunity for a stepwise illness adaptation. Psychosocial impairment may result from aphasic communication deficits (e.g. social withdrawal because of communicative incompetence), but also may have a negative effect upon language skills (e.g. by lack of social and communicative contacts).

III Neurobehavioral disorders may directly (e.g. by reducing the patient's and his/her family's mobility) or indirectly (e.g. by causing apractic disorders) and hereby influencing nonverbal (compensatory) communicative means influence the psychosocial condition.

In the following, psychosocial changes in aphasic patients will be considered with respect to the following domains:

- professional,
- social,
- familial and,
- psychological alterations.

PROFESSIONAL CHANGES

The structure of insurance and social security systems differs widely between different countries, so that comparative analyses of professional changes resulting from aphasia are difficult. With few exceptions, patients suffering from chronic aphasia are not professionally reintegrated[27]. Besides their advanced age and the inflexibility of the job market to employ residual intact capacities, the instantness of stroke precludes gradual adaptations and compensations with respect to professional performance[28].

The vast majority of aphasics have to retire. Matsumoto et al.[35] reported that 33% of stroke victims, but only 3% of aphasics retained employment. Retirement leads to social changes (loss of social contacts, role change within the family by losing the role of breadwinner).

SOCIAL CHANGES

Social isolation, deprivation, and changes in social status have been reported as frequent social consequences of aphasia. Buck[6] emphasized that aphasia does not only affect the social role of the patient, but also to a considerable extent the social condition of his/her family.

Joussen and Pascher[27] conducted a survey for social changes in 25 unselected aphasics. Their subjects complained about social isolation and downward social mobility. Commonly, the patient's family shares social isolation: Artes and Hoops[2] reported that more than 40% of the wives of aphasics felt socially isolated in comparison to only every sixth spouse of non-aphasic brain damaged patients.

FAMILIAL CHANGES

Buck[6] described aphasia as a "family illness." The wives of aphasics complain about intrafamilial tension, loss of partnership, and severely impaired sexual relations[28]. They feel strained by having to take over tasks and decisions that previously had been the aphasics' responsibility and react with aggression or depression[34]. Kinsella and Duffy[29] reported that two out of five spouses suffer from a clinical degree of depression and four out of five take tranquilizers or sedatives.

Frustration of the aphasic may lead to anger of the spouse, rejection, and break-down of communication between the partners[36]. Such problems and maladjustments tend to increase with time[28]. With respect to their children and their education, aphasic patients complain about loss of authority resulting from their communication impairment[5].

Malone[33] pointed out that these intrafamilial tensions are enhanced by "unhealthy attitudes" on the side of the relatives such as hyperprotection, rejection, or denial of impairment[28]. Relatives' unrealistic estimations concerning communicative abilities and future improvements have been reported by Helmick et al.[16] and Müller et al.[39]. Oranen et al.[41] described various patterns of familial coping with the best adjusted families exhibiting an optimistic coping approach. Depressive or nervous approaches were related with inadequate adjustment.

PSYCHOLOGICAL CHANGES

In the last decade, depressive mood changes following stroke gained importance both for our understanding of the mechanisms underlying impairment and for rehabilitation. Despite intensive research, the published results and conclusions of studies investigating etiology and pathogenesis of depressive symptoms in aphasic patients vary greatly. Lipsey et al.[32] reported "clinically significant depression" to occur in 30 to 60% of patients suffering from brain infarction, whereas House et al.[25] reported figures of 11% one month and 5% one year post stroke. Comparisons of the various studies are hampered by differences in patient selection, use of different instruments for the assessment of depressive changes, and, most of all, differences in the underlying pathogenetic concepts.

Mainly three concepts have been advanced:

1) Aphasic stroke may result in a depressive disorder as defined by standard psychiatric classification systems[44].

2) "(Depressive-) catastrophic reactions" constitute a class of emotional-affective reactions that are specific for brain-damaged patients[3,12].
3) The depressive reaction following stroke is a natural "grief response"[50]. Benson[4] went so far as to state that the reactive depression was a "... healthy sign, indicating sufficient recovery of intellectual competency for recognition of the severity of the problem and the subsequent alterations in life style" (p.176).

In a series of studies, Robinson, Starkstein, and collaborators were able to establish the following:

- major depressive disorders are a frequent and often neglected or underestimated consequence of cerebrovascular insults with aphasia[44,49];
- they may be present in the acute phase and usually last for one to two years[43];
- presence and degree of mood disorders correlate negatively with success of rehabilitation[42];
- depressive changes are more frequent with left hemisphere lesions and their degree correlates with lesion localization[48].

These data indicate that at least a relevant proportion of post-stroke depressive disorders is anatomically determined and that mood disorders are relevant with respect to outcome of rehabilitation.

We[24] investigated depressive changes in 21 acute and 21 chronic aphasic patients with single left sided stroke lesions, who had no previous history of psychiatric disorder or alcohol abuse, using an observer rating scale for depression ("*Cornell Scale for Depression*"[1]), the RDC classification[47] for the diagnosis of major or minor depressive disorder, and other instruments. There were no significant differences with respect to overall depression scores between the two groups. Neither age, sex, degree of hemiparesis, nor lesion volume discriminated the patients with respect to presence and degree of depressive symptoms. In the acute but not in the chronic group, nonfluency of speech production correlated with the severity of depressive changes. Only in the acute group, six patients could be identified who corresponded to the RDC-criteria of "major depression." Their mood disorder could not be interpreted as an artifact of the in-patient condition and corresponded to the symptomatology found in endogenous major depression.

Based on the data of different studies of psychosocial alterations in aphasic patients and their families[20,21]; Wenz & Herrmann[55] proposed a three stage interactive pathogenetic model for depressive changes in stroke patients[22,23] (Figure 11–2). In our opinion it seems to be more adequate to consider depressive changes as dependent on illness course-oriented rehabilitation stages, rather than to distinguish dichotomous categories such as purely reactive or "endogeneous" depression. In each stage of illness and rehabilitation the aphasic patient has a specific vulnerability (based on various causes) to develop mood disorders.

In the acute and early postacute primary stage of rehabilitation, depression seems to be mainly of the endogenous type and caused by direct structural and biochemical consequences of stroke. In the second stage that roughly corresponds to the clinical rehabilitation period two to six months post stroke, psychoreactive mood changes following the realization of neurological and neuropsychological dysfunctions (and their possibly long standing duration) come to the fore. Besides persisting endogeneous factors, reactive components could have a new or additional impact on the development of depression. Finally, in the third, chronic stage when the patient is discharged from in-patient treatment, depression could result from realizing the whole scope of professional, intrafamilial, and social alterations produced by lasting impairment.

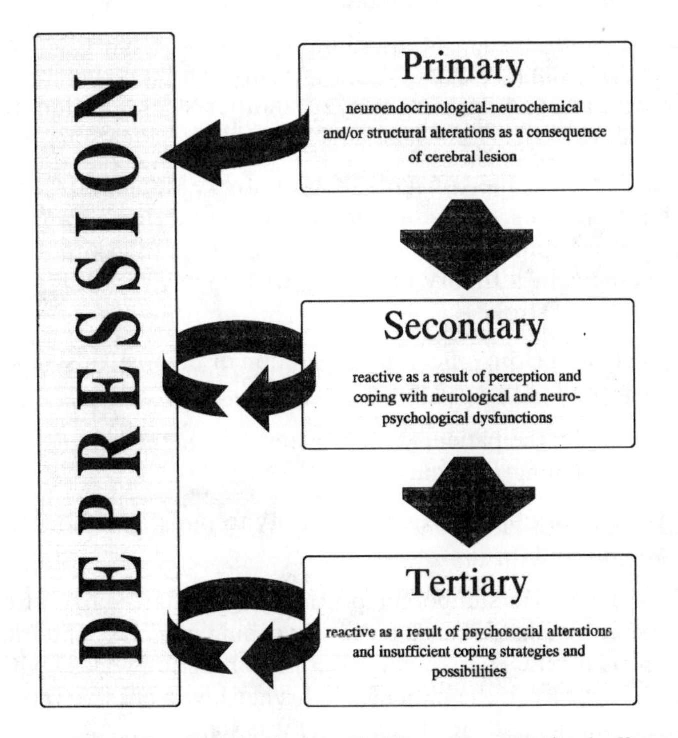

Different Aspects of Vulnerability to Depressive Changes in a Multi-Time and Factor Model (based on Herrmann et al.[23]).

Figure 11–2

The term "catastrophic reaction" was coined by Goldstein[13,14] to describe a class of emotional reactions specific for brain damaged patients. Gainotti[12] (p.44) distinguished depressive mood changes and indifference reactions from catastrophic reactions upon the effects of brain damage and described the latter category of behaviors to include the following: anxiety reaction, tears, aggressive behavior, swears, displacement, refusal, renouncement, and compensatory boasting. To avoid confusion these reactions should not be used synonymous with depression but regarded as a different entity of mood changes[49]. Gainotti reported a higher incidence of these emotional "catastrophic" reactions in aphasic than in non-aphasic brain damaged patients. Quite characteristically, these behaviors are exhibited after communicative failure:

> "With mounting feelings of frustration and depression, and then of hostility, the patient, rather suddenly during testing or treatment, breaks into laboured sobbing and weeping, often accompanied by phrases, sounds or gestures which indicate both hopelessness and anger. The anger is directed toward the examiner, and the patient refuses to carry on with any language procedure or even with simple conversation"[3] (p.56).

Charatan and Fisk[7] stressed the importance of fears for the emotional reactions in stroke patients, especially fears of being left permanently crippled and handicapped, of another stroke, of impoverishment, of loss of love. (It must be added that all these fears are realistic.)

In contrast to the concepts of post-stroke depression and catastrophic reactions, the concept of "grief-reaction" or "grief-response"[50,51] is explicitly psychodynamical and tries to incorporate these mood changes in a theory of coping with losses resulting from the consequences of stroke:

- the loss of close others (by separation or divorce, or symbolically by lack of personal contact),
- the loss of the patient's self or identity (e.g., the loss of psychic or physical integrity), and
- the loss of objects (e.g. the inability to pursue previous hobbies and interests).

Tanner and Gerstenberger postulate a regular course of coping with these losses that is based on earlier coping models[30]. Intensity and duration of its stages may vary, but "the reactions occur with predictable regularity in the patient and his/her loved ones"[51] (p.81). According to Tanner and Gerstenberger, these stages are:

- Denial of the neurological and neuropsychological sequelae, that may be complete, partial, passive, and mystical ("I have a significant speech and language disorder, but it is temporary; God will make me whole again", p.81), or existential (the patient is convinced to overcome his deficits by his own resources).

- Frustration, commonly combined with fear.
- Depression, in response to the realization that the consequences of the stroke are irreversible. Occasional euphorical episodes are interpreted by Tanner and Gerstenberger as regressions to the denial stage.
- Acceptance: "Acceptance is the goal of grieving; it is the light at the end of the tunnel"[51] (p.83).

Although the logical consistency of Tanner's and Gerstenberger's concept and its relation to the results and theories of research into coping with the consequences of extracerebral disease may be appealing, two criticisms must be raised:

- the psychodynamic concept negates the wealth of findings concerning the role of the specific depressive disorders that are present at least in subgroups of stroke victims;
- the concept offers hardly any therapeutic implications and may lead to de-emphasizing the patient's strain:

> "Somehow it must be felt that if a therapist is able to 'stage' a patient's response to catastrophe, then the patient's responses become more understandable/manageable, because they can be interpreted as taking place within a theoretical context"[15] (p.85).

PSYCHOSOCIAL CHANGES WITH APHASIA

As Code and Müller[8] have pointed out, the psychosocial perspective is the most underdeveloped aspect in the rehabilitation process:

> "Psychosocial adjustment concerns not only coming to terms with a totally new set of circumstances for the individual experiencing aphasia, but has wider implications within the social network in which the individual lives, and in particular on the family. The prime focus of research into psychosocial adjustment is to understand better how to facilitate psychological well-being in aphasic individuals; the effects an aphasic individual has on significant others and implications for the family and the broader social network; and the extent to which society in its broadest sense is able to respond and accommodate these changes in a positive manner"[37].

The above review of the literature has demonstrated that psychosocial changes following aphasic stroke affect professional, social, familial, and psychological aspects of the life of the patient as well as his/her family. In a survey of 20 chronic, severely nonfluent aphasics, their closest others, and their therapists, Herrmann and Wallesch attempted to quantify and compare:

- the various psychosocial burdens related with aphasia using the approach of Weissman and Paykel[54] to assess the degree of changes through applying ratings to statements, and
- the expectations of patients, relatives, and therapists concerning future improvement and adjustment using the Code-Müller Scale of Psychosocial Adjustment[9,38,39].

The rating scale for psychosocial changes included the following categories:

0: No change in comparison to premorbid performance/ability.

1: minor changes which rarely and only mildly affect everyday life.

2: changes are noticed from time to time and then affect the patient and his social environment.

3: changes are frequently noticed and have an impact upon everyday life.

4: changes are noticed permanently, are a burden for the family's everyday life, and cannot be compensated.

The four classes of psychological, professional, familial, and social changes were rated as affecting everyday life to a similar extent by the aphasic's relatives. Figures 11–3 to 11–6 show the results for the various items presented to the patient's relatives.

The psychosocial alterations experienced by the patients' relatives were manifold and were rated as affecting the families' everyday life to a considerable extent. Changes in 'professional' abilities included even simple household tasks. Eighty per cent of the patients were unable to maintain their premorbid domestic responsibilities and tasks. Social contacts related to the patient's job had worn thin, only in four cases they were rated as little or not impaired. A number of relatives reported that there had been efforts to re-establish these contacts, which in most instances had been rejected by the former workmates.

The relatives acknowledged financial burdens resulting from the patient's illness and a downward progression of the standard of living in most instances. The extreme rating (a permanent burden that cannot be compensated) was not used with respect to the family's financial condition, which is probably due to the German social security and pension system that provides adequate support for those persons that have had employment for more than 15 years. The necessity to care for the patient frequently prevented the relatives from contributing to the household income.

Psychosocial changes as rated by the relatives of 20 chronic nonfluent aphasics (data from Herrmann & Wallesch[20]; for rating categories, see text).

Figures 11–3 to 11–6

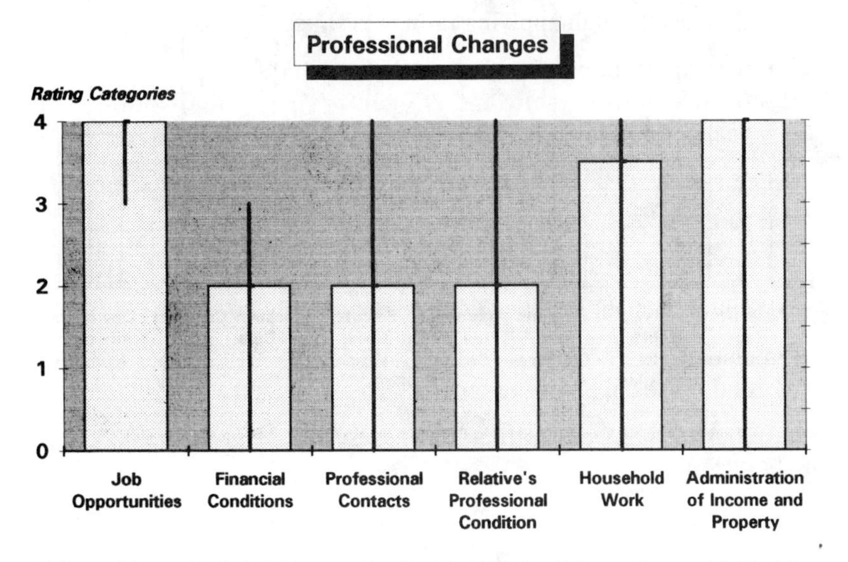

Medians and Ranges of Professional Changes as Rated by Patients' Relatives (data from Herrmann & Wallesch[20])

Figure 11–3

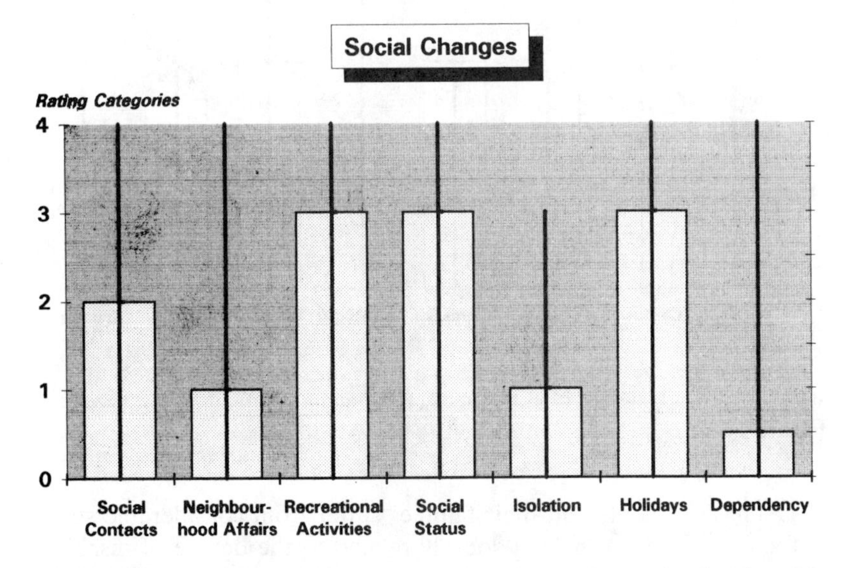

Medians and Ranges of Social Changes as Rated by Patients' Relatives (data from Herrmann & Wallesch[20])

Figure 11–4

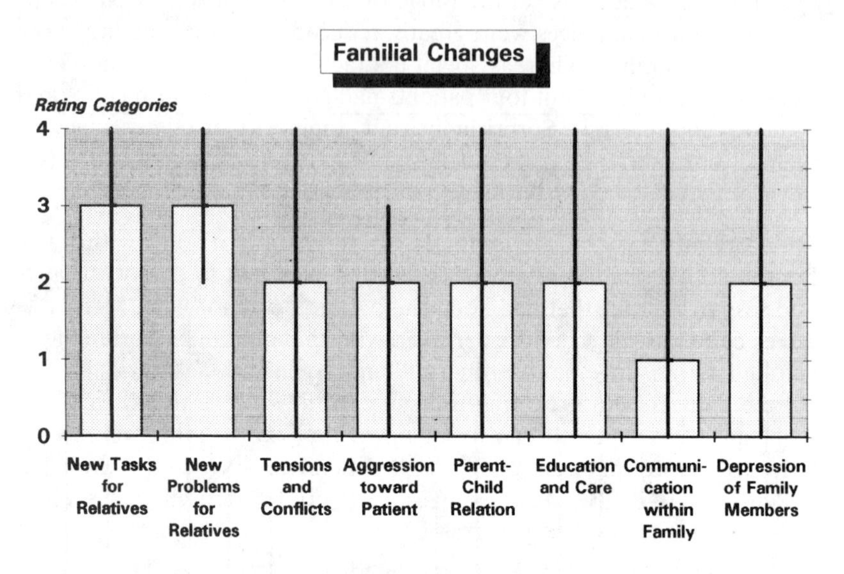

Medians and Ranges of Familial Changes as Rated by Patients' Relatives (data from Herrmann & Wallesch[20])
Figure 11–5

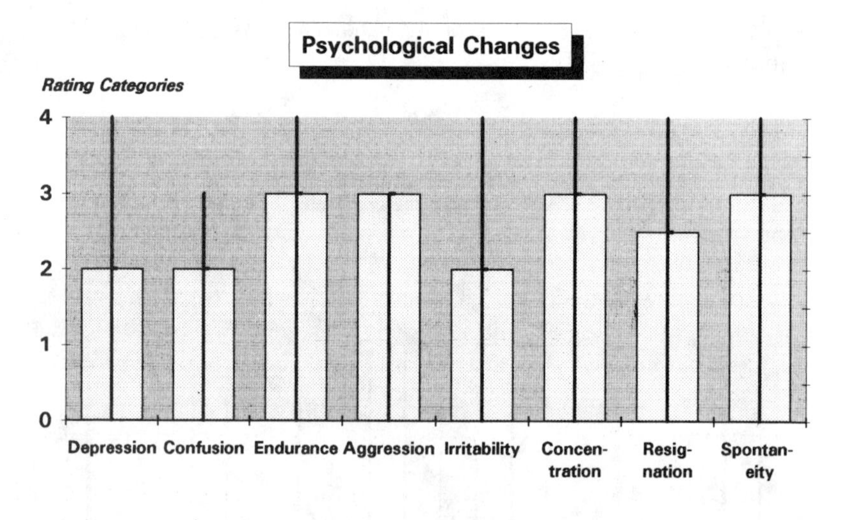

Medians and Ranges of Psychological Changes as Rated by Patients' Relatives (data from Herrmann & Wallesch[20])
Figure 11–6

Aphasic patients and their families suffer from considerable social restrictions. These were only loosely related to the degree of disability and rather indicate social stigmatization ("disabled family"). The relatives reported a decrease of the range of social interactions: Contacts to friends and acquantances were greatly reduced or had ceased in almost half of the families, whereas social contacts with neighbors remained rather unaffected. All but four patients had given up former recreational activities and interests. Surprisingly, only a minority of relatives viewed themselves as suffering from social isolation. Three years post stroke (on the average), they may have adapted to the altered social circumstances.

Familial changes are dominated by a change of roles within the household. Almost all relatives stated that they had to deal with tasks and responsibilities that had been the patient's premorbidly. Many relatives complained of being overtaxed with the additional workload resulting from management of financial and organizational affairs, caring for the aphasic, and providing transport to the various treatments. Female spouses frequently had to delegate their own premorbid household tasks. Fifty per cent of the family members included in the Hermann and Wallesch study complained about depression or feeling lonely, which they interpreted as resulting from being over-taxed and physically and mentally exhausted.

Communication within the family was not viewed as a relevant problem by most relatives. In almost all cases, the family was able to adapt communication strategies and establish a sufficient degree of communication on issues of everyday life by non- and paraverbal means on the side of the patient and by altered communication behavior of the other family members[18,19].

Psychological changes in the aphasics, especially depression, resignation, helplessness, and despair, were noted by almost all the relatives and interpreted as a reaction to the disability. The question "Does the patient exhibit aggressiveness or anger towards his impairment, himself, or others?" was agreed upon by 85% of relatives. Manifest use of violence against wheelchair, prosthesis, or paretic extremities was frequently mentioned. The comparatively high incidence of this type of behavior in our study was viewed as related to the patients' relatively severe impairment in comparison to other studies.

EXPECTATIONS FOR PSYCHOSOCIAL ADJUSTMENT

In the second part of our above mentioned study, we investigated patients', relatives', and (mainly speech) therapists' expectations concerning future psychosocial adjustment. We used a revised Code-Müller Scale[9,38] that consists of ten questions such as "Do you think the ability to meet friends socially ...?" and five rating categories:

0: will become much worse

1: will deteriorate a bit

2: will remain unchanged

3: will improve a bit

4: will improve much.

An "optimism score"[39] was calculated as the sum of the individual scores assigned to the 10 items of the Code-Müller scale.

Patients and relatives expected significant improvement with respect to speech skills and being able to cope with embarrassment due to speech problems, the relatives in addition hoped for improvement in independence, depression, and frustration. The therapists expected no significant improvement, but rather feared deterioration in social capabilities such as forming new personal relationships. The optimism scores of the therapists were significantly lower than those of patients and relatives (see Herrmann & Wallesch[21], for a criticism of the comparative value of the Code-Müller scale as it was used in the 1989 study).

This difference in expectations may pose an obstacle to the conduct and goals of rehabilitation treatment. With few exceptions, the primary goals of rehabilitation of chronic, severely nonfluent aphasics would be to optimize the use of residual capacities and to consolidate therapeutic achievements. This strategy is opposed to the expectations of future improvement that were expressed by patients and their relatives.

Most patients included in the Herrmann and Wallesch[20] study had been under our care in the acute or early postacute stage. At that time, they had received information concerning etiology, type of impairment, and prognosis. However, when interviewed for the investigation, a majority of relatives complained about not having received sufficient information, especially none about how to care for and how to communicate with the aphasic partner. A considerable number of relatives had hopes — even after years of very limited progress — that the premorbid levels of functions and abilities would be eventually restored. These inappropriate expectations result in emotional and motivational crises that are damaging both for the intrafamilial and therapeutical interactions. The data of Johannsen-Horbach et al.[26] suggest that information concerning disease, disabilities and their consequences should repeatedly be offered in the chronic stage, when the relatives are actually confronted with these issues.

Numerous studies have established that the attitude and cooperation of the family members exert a positive influence upon the process and results of rehabilitation[10,11,31,52]. Johannsen-Horbach et al.[26] warn against assigning the role of a "co-therapist" to the spouse because of the additional effect to the disadvantage of the aphasic on the balance of powers within the familiy. Rehabilitation approaches that include family members should therefore focus on measures of tertiary prevention, i.e. reduction and prevention of late and secondary sequelae of manifest impairments. These aims can only be accomplished by inclusion or separate counselling of the patient's family members[20,26].

EMOTIONAL REACTIONS AND ILLNESS PERCEPTION IN CHRONIC APHASIA

Therapy focusing on tertiary prevention that includes the patient and his/her relatives presupposes an agreement on the relevant symptoms and disabilities. However, aphasics and their relatives disagree as to which symptoms are the greatest burdens. Wenz and Herrmann[55] investigated emotional reactions and illness perception in 10 chronic aphasics and one relative of each patient. They found only little correlation between subjective impairment and emotional strain in both groups. The aphasics considered their hemiparesis as the most relevant symptom (44% of the total impairment caused by disease symptoms as compared to 29% in the view of the relatives). The relatives rated non-aphasic neuropsychological impairment markedly higher than the patients (21% vs. 12%). Both agreed on the limited relative impact of language impairment (aphasics: 27%, relatives: 29%).

In the view of the aphasics, emotional strain was mainly caused by changes in job opportunities and the impairment of talking to strangers. Their partnership was experienced as giving emotional relief. The relatives, on the other hand, reported emotional strain mainly to result from their own depression and the aphasic's inability to express his wishes and feelings within the family. Not surprisingly in view of the different emotional perceptions, patients and relatives differed in their views with respect to familial changes. The aphasics experienced their family as stable (7% of illness related social and psychological alterations), whereas the relatives reported marked intrafamilial changes (20%).

THERAPEUTIC IMPLICATIONS

The psychosocial perspective in aphasia therapy is the most underdeveloped and yet is fundamental in the rehabilitation process[8]. As has been outlined, the aphasic and his/her relatives suffer from various and partially incongruous psychosocial burdens and may hold unrealistic expectations that interfere with the goals of traditional training therapy. Burdens and expectations are both targets for psychosocially and psychotherapeutically oriented treatment approaches. Inclusion of relatives into the treatment of the aphasic has been suggested and opposed (for a review, see Johannsen-Horbach et al.[26]). In many instances, both the aphasic patient and his/her relatives require psychotherapeutic counseling or treatment. Under the WHO[56] definition, the relatives suffer from a disease-related handicap affecting their psychological and social well-being.

The different perceptions of the relevance of symptoms and the emotional strain they cause should preclude treatment of aphasic and relative in the same session, unless these issues have been considered and therapeutically approached. We consider traditional family therapy[40,45,53] a psychotherapeutic technique of questionable value for the treatment of psychosocial strains in families that include an aphasic. Herrmann[17] expressed doubts as to whether such family system can be adequately described and interpreted within the framework of traditional family therapy. However, we agree that strategies taken from family therapy may be used for crisis intervention when aphasia is acute or an acute crisis is present[40].

Our present approach is to treat aphasics and relatives separately. In our opinion none of the major psychotherapeutic techniques is able to cope with a patient who is deprived of his central means of communication. In aphasics of advanced age who live in stable social and familial circumstances and who have had some rewards in their premorbid life, we have made positive experiences with a psychosocially oriented group approach[26]. This type of treatment failed with younger patients. For relatives, we propose an open, non-directive, client centered approach. We had positive preliminary results with a relatives' group following these lines[26].

SUMMARY

Psychosocial consequences of aphasia exceed communication impairment. The aphasic patients and their relatives interviewed by Wenz and Herrmann[55] considered language disability to contribute less than 30% to their overall burden. Emotional strain was mainly caused by social and psychosocial alterations, within the family in the relatives' view, and mainly concerning external social relations in the opinion of the aphasics.

The following domains of relevant psychosocial alterations were reviewed:

- professional changes
- social changes
- familial changes
- psychological changes.

Whereas in the acute stage, the depression of the aphasic appears to have an organic basis, the psychopathological consequences in the chronic stage both for the aphasic and his/her relatives are mainly reactive. These reactions of aphasic and relatives are not congruent. The divergence in strategies and goals of coping may form a major obstacle for rehabilitation. In our opinion, the evaluation of psychotherapeutic strategies for brain damaged patients and their relatives aiming at psychosocial impairment and coping with the direct and indirect consequences of disability is a major goal for future rehabilitation research.

REFERENCES

1. Alexopoulos, G.S., Abrams, R.C., Young, R.C. & Shamoian, C.A.(1988): Use of the Cornell Scale in nondemented patients. *J Am Geriat Soc.,* **36:** 230–236.
2. Artes, R. & Hoops, R.(1976): Problems of aphasic and nonaphasic stroke patients as identified and evaluated by patients' wives, **in** Lebrun, Y., Hoops, R. (eds.): *Recovery in Aphasics.* Amsterdam: Swets & Zeitlinger.
3. Benson, D.F. (1973): Psychiatric aspects of aphasia. *Brit J Psychiat.,* **123:** 555–566.
4. Benson, D.F.(1979): Psychiatric aspects of aphasia, **in** Benson, D.F.(ed.): *Aphasia, Alexia and Agraphia.* New York: Churchill Livingstone.
5. Biorn-Hansen, V. (1957): Social and emotional aspects of aphasia. *J Speech Hear Dis.,* **22:** 52–59.
6. Buck, M. (1968): *Dysphasia. Professional guide for family and patient.* Englewood Cliffs: Prentice Hall.
7. Charatan, F.B. & Fisk, A. (1978): The mental and emotional results of stroke. *N.Y. State J Med.,* **78:** 1403–1405.
8. Code, C. & Müller, D.J. (1983): Perspectives in aphasia therapy, **in** Code, C. & Müller, D.J. (eds.): *Aphasia therapy.* London: Arnold.
9. Code, C. & Müller, D.J. (in press): The Code-Müller protocols: Assessing perceptions of psychosocial adjustment to aphasia. Kibworth: Far Communications.
10. Derman, S., Manaster, A. (1967): Family counselling with relatives of aphasic patients at Schwab rehabilitation hospital. *ASHA,* **9:** 175–177.
11. Florance, C.(1979): The aphasic's significant other: Training and counseling, **in** Brookshire, R.(ed.), *Clinical Aphasiology Conference Proceedings.* Minneapolis: BRK.
12. Gainotti, G.(1972): Emotional behaviour and hemispheric side of the lesion. *Cortex,* **8:** 41–55.
13. Goldstein, K.(1939): *The organism: A holistic approach to biology derived from pathological data in man.* New York: American Book Company.
14. Goldstein, K.(1948): *Language and language disturbances.* New York: Grune & Stratton.
15. Gordon, W.A., Hibbard, M.R. & Morganstein, S.(1988): Response to Tanner and Gerstenberger. *Aphasiology,* **2:** 85–88.
16. Helmick, J.W., Watamori, T.S. & Palmer, J.M. (1976): Spouses' understanding of the communication disabilities of aphasic patients. *J. Speech Hear Dis.,* **41:** 238–243.
17. Herrmann, M.(1989): On the possible value of family therapy in aphasia rehabilitation. *Aphasiology,* **3:** 491–492.
18. Herrmann, M., Koch, U., Johannsen-Horbach, H. & Wallesch, C.W.(1989): Communicative skills in chronic and severe nonfluent aphasia. *Brain & Language,* **37:** 339–352.
19. Herrmann, M., Reichle, T., Lucius-Hoene, G., Wallesch, C.W. & Johannsen-Horbach, H. (1988): Nonverbal communication as a compensative strategy for severely nonfluent aphasics — A quantitative approach. *Brain & Language,* **33:** 41–54.
20. Herrmann, M. & Wallesch, C.W. (1989): Psychosocial changes and psychosocial adjustment with chronic and severe nonfluent aphasia. *Aphasiology,* **3:** 513–526.

21. Herrmann, M. & Wallesch, C.W. (1990): Expectations of psychosocial adjustment in aphasia: a MAUT study with the Code-Müller Scale of Psychosocial Ajustment. *Aphasiology,* **4:** 527–538.
22. Herrmann, M. (1991): *Emotional-affektive Veränderungen nach cerebrovaskulären Insulten mit Aphasie.* University of Freiburg: Med.Diss.
23. Herrmann, M., Bartels, C. & Wallesch, C.W. (in press): Depression und Aphasie — Konzepte zur Ätiopathogenese und Implikationen für Forschung und Rehabilitation. *Neurolinguistik.*
24. Herrmann, M., Bartels, C. & Wallesch, C.W. (submitted): Depression in acute and chronic aphasia: Symptoms, pathoanatomical-clinical correlations and functional implications.
25. House, A., Dennis, M., Warlow, C., Hawton, K. & Molyneux, A.(1990): Mood disorders after stroke and their relation to lesion location: A CT-scan study. *Brain,* **113:** 1113–1129.
26. Johannsen-Horbach, H., Wenz, C., Fünfgeld, M., Herrmann, M. & Wallesch, C.W. (in press): Psychosocial aspects in the treatment of adult aphasics and their families — A group approach. **In:** Holland, A. & Forbes, M. (eds.): *World perspectives on aphasia.* San Diego: Singular.
27. Joussen, K. & Pascher, W. (1984): Empirische Untersuchungen der sozialen Situation von Aphasikern. *Folia Phoniatrica,* **36:** 66–73.
28. Kinsella, G., & Duffy, F.D. (1978): The spouse of the aphasic patient, **in** Lebrun,Y. & Hoops,R. (eds.): *The management of aphasia.* Amsterdam: Swets & Zetlinger.
29. Kinsella, G. & Duffy, F.D. (1979): Psychosocial readjustment in the spouses of aphasic patients. *Scand J Rehab Med.,* **11:** 129–132.
30. Kübler-Ross, E. (1969): *On death and dying.* New York: Macmillan.
31. Lesser, R., Bryan, K., Anderson, J. & Hilton, R.(1986): Involving relatives in aphasia therapy: an application of language enrichment therapy. *Int J Rehab Res.,* **9:** 259–267.
32. Lipsey, J.R., Robinson, R.G., Pearlyon, G.D., Rao, K. & Price, T.R. (1985): The dexamethasone suppression test and mood following stroke. *Am J Psychiat.,* **142:** 318–323.
33. Malone, R.L. (1969): Expressed attitudes of families of aphasics. *J Speech Hear Dis.,* **24:** 146–151.
34. Malone, R., Ptacek, P. & Malone, M.(1970): Attitudes expressed by families of aphasics. *Brit J Dis Comm.,* **5:** 174–179.
35. Matsumoto, N., Whisnant, J.P., Kurland, L.T. & Okasaki, H. (1973): Natural history of stroke in Rochester, Minnesota, 1955–1969: An extension of a previous study, 1945 through 1954. *Stroke,* **4:** 20–29.
36. Mulhall, D.J. (1978): Dysphasic stroke patients and the influence of their relatives. *Brit J Dis Comm.,* **13:** 127–134.
37. Müller, D.J. (1992): Psychosocial aspects of aphasia, **in** Blanken, G., Dittmann, J., Grimm, H., Marshall, J.C. and Wallesch, C.W.(eds.): *Linguistic Disorders and Pathologies.* Berlin: De Gruyter.
38. Müller, D.J. & Code, C. (1983): Interpersonal perceptions of psychosocial adjustment to aphasia, **in** Code, C. and Müller, D.J.(eds.): *Aphasia therapy.* London: Arnold.
39. Müller, D.J., Code, C., Mugford, J. (1983): Predicting psychosocial adjustment to aphasia. *Brit J Dis Comm.,* **18:** 23–29.
40. Norlin, P.F.(1986): Familiar faces, sudden strangers: Helping families cope with the crisis of aphasia, **in** Chapey, R.(ed.): *Language intervention strategies in adult aphasia* (2nd ed.). Baltimore: Williams & Wilkins.
41. Oranen, M., Sihvonen, R., Aysto, S. & Hagfors, C.(1987): Different coping patterns in the families of aphasic people. *Aphasiology,* **1:** 277–281.
42. Parikh, R.M., Robinson, R.G., Lipsey, J.R. & Starkstein, S.E. (1990): The impact of poststroke depression on recovery in activities of daily living over a two-year follow-up. *Archives of Neurology,* **47:** 785–789.
43. Robinson, R.G., Bolduc, P.L. & Price, T.R. (1987): Two-year longitudinal study of poststroke mood disorders: Comparison of acute-onset with delayed-onset depression. *Am J Psychiat.,* **143:** 1238–1244.

44. Robinson, R.G. & Starkstein, S.E.(1990): Current research in affective disorders following stroke. *J Neuropsychiat Clin Neurosci.*, **2:** 1–14.
45. Rollin, W.J. (1984): Family therapy and the aphasic adult, **in** Eisenson, J.(ed.): *Adult aphasia* (2nd ed.) Englewood Cliffs: Prentice Hall.
46. Schwab, J.J. (1972): Emotional considerations in cancer and stroke. *NY State J Med.*, **72:** 2877–2880.
47. Spitzer, R.L., Endicott, J. & Robins, E.(1975): *Research diagnostic criteria (RDC) for a group of functional disorders.* New York: Psychiatric Institute.
48. Starkstein, S.E., Robinson, R.G. & Price, T.R.(1987): Comparison of cortical and subcortical lesions in the production of poststroke mood disorders. *Brain,* **110:** 1045–1059.
49. Starkstein, S.E. & Robinson, R.G. (1988): Aphasia and depression. *Aphasiology,* **2:** 1–20.
50. Tanner, D.C.(1980): Loss and grief: Implications for the speech-language pathologist and audiologist. *J Am Speech Hear Ass.,* **22:** 916–928.
51. Tanner, D.C. & Gerstenberger, D.L.(1988): The grief response in neuropathologies of speech and language. *Aphasiology,* **2:** 79–84.
52. Turnblom, M. & Myers, J.S.(1952): Group discussion programs with the families of aphasic patients. *J Speech Hear Dis.,* **17:** 393–396.
53. Währborg, P.(1989): Aphasia and family therapy. *Aphasiology,* **3:** 479–482.
54. Weissman, K. & Paykel, E.S. (1974): *The depressed woman.* Chicago: University of Chicago Press.
55. Wenz, C. & Herrmann, M. (1990): Emotionales Erleben und subjektive Krankheitswahrnehmung bei chronischer Aphasia—ein Vergleich zwischen Patienten und deren Familienangehörigen. Psychother. *Psychosom med Psychol.,* **40:** 488–495.
56. World Health Organization (1980): *International classification of impairments, disabilities, and handicaps.* Geneva: WHO.

CHAPTER 12

THE PERSON WITH APHASIA AND SOCIETY

M.-A. LEMAY

THE PERSON WITH APHASIA AND SOCIETY

THE PERSON WITH APHASIA AND SOCIETY

The very title of this chapter attests to the inherent estrangement between the person with aphasia and the *rest of society*; is the person or society to blame? (undoubtedly both are partly responsible). This gap can be perceived as a division into two camps, two opposing teams, each of which is attempting to decode the other's strategies.

Society is healthy and hale: People gulp down their breakfast and bustle off to work. They can easily cope with traffic jams and overcrowded subways it is all part of everyday life. Work is fraught with discussions with colleagues, decisions to be made, telephone calls to clients, letters to be written, and instructions to be carried out. Then comes lunch break — prime time for a brief excursion to the bank or to a store to pick up an item. Finally, it is time to go home and reimmerse oneself in family life: New discussions, minor problems to solve, and more decisions. The children's homework must be checked, the babysitter must be contacted, family reunions must be planned, and the bills must be paid. Yet few people become exhausted from this daily marathon! Granted, it is somewhat tiring, but one can always relax in front of the television. Soon enough, it will be vacation time. Oh yes! Don't forget to confirm the reservations, another call to add to tomorrow's list.

In this daily runaround, the brain ponders, reasons, memorizes, decides, calculates, and decodes and produces endless messages. The body, too, acts —moving, eating, or resting. All this nothing more than a typical everyday routine. Who can imagine for a moment that a simple phone call to an insurance agent or a regular day of grocery shopping can be transformed overnight into a devastating nightmare, if not an Olympic-scale challenge which is relived each and every day?

The world of the person with aphasia is a limited one. During the long months immediately after the stroke, health care, rest, appointments, and therapy sessions come to occupy the time that was formerly devoted to work, sports, social gatherings, leisure, and reading. A new routine emerges, one which is largely beyond the person's control. The persons' acceptance of their situation is linked to the promise of recovery, and also to the fact that they now lack the energy to make decisions on their own.

Communication: Making Oneself Heard

Language enables one to carve out one's place in society, and to achieve recognition as an individual. Consequently, the verbal impairment, more than the motor disability, remains the most difficult for persons with aphasia to accept. How can these persons make themselves heard when they cannot clearly express their ideas, opinions, and perceptions of things and events because the vocabulary and phrases which convey nuances and add precision to normal conversation are no longer at their disposal? Persons with aphasia sometimes barely succeed in expressing even the most basic needs. Here is one testimony from a person with aphasia regarding the difficulties he experienced during the acute phase of his illness.

> "I was in the hospital. I couldn't speak. They wanted to feed me, but I didn't want to eat. I wanted milk. They didn't give me any. That made me angry. I wanted to go home. I wanted to make a phone call, but I couldn't."[1]

The language impairment is aggravated by its far-reaching consequences on all aspects of cultural life. The person with aphasia often can no longer read, write, nor calculate, and he may substitute inappropriate words instead of the intended words; for example, saying "Hello Sir" to a woman, or saying "my mother" instead of "my wife." These difficulties may lead observers in society to question the person's intellectual capacities. Persons with aphasia feel divested of the cultural baggage which they previously possessed — that which makes up the foundation of their personality. Mrs. S. exclaims, "You are completely transformed, it isn't you any more."

Most persons with aphasia must complacently accept the role of the listener when they find themselves in a group, because they can no longer actively participate in a conversation. They would like to contribute, but words escape them, and the topic changes too quickly. One patient reports:

> "I was a man who used to talk a lot, about many things. Before, I used to make jokes. No more. The words don't come quick enough."

In his *Portrait of Aphasia* [(6)], David Knox reports that his wife, once she acquired aphasia, attributed her social isolation to her inability to contribute normally to a conversation with an individual or a group. She considered this feeling of being an outsider the change in her life that was the most difficult to accept. Naturally, she was eventually able to adapt with fair success, but she will never truly accept her condition.

In order for persons with aphasia to consider themselves viable partners in a conversation, they must feel integrated. They need to be speakers whose opinions are solicited, along with information about events, people, procedures, or decisions. They will then experience an authentic *exchange,* the only worthy dialogue in their view.

---

[1] This testimony, as well as the other quotes below, were gathered from personal interviews with persons with aphasia that were conducted for this chapter.

Paradoxically, persons with aphasia, at least at the onset of this new consuming experience, tend to flee from communication opportunities, out of the constant fear of making mistakes, "saying silly things," to quote one person with aphasia. In fact, misunderstandings are quite common; some arise from inappropriate words which sometimes throw *listeners* off the track, if they neglect to take the context into account. Other misunderstandings occur when the *person with aphasia* misinterprets the speaker's message. In this case, the speaker will also become frustrated because of the disruption in the verbal exchange. He may have difficulty coping with the constant effort to mentally and orally fill in the words omitted by the person with aphasia along with hesitations, errors, and words which can mean virtually anything: *Close the window* may mean *close the door, draw the curtains,* or even *open the window.* If the family eventually adjusts and does succeed in decoding this novel use of language, friends and outsiders do not always have the time and patience necessary to do so. Initial encouragement and particular (at times patronizing) consideration by others soon gives way to excuses to justify the retreat spurred by growing discomfort.

Isolation

An extensive study[7] conducted in the United States in 1986 featuring 1,665 neurological patients (without specifying which hemisphere was damaged), reported that persons with strokes tended to be more functional in the activities of daily living (ADL) than in social interaction. Although these patients were slightly more dependent in ADL when they lived with someone, in that case they scored comparatively higher (on an evaluation scale) in social interaction. Notwithstanding numerous extraneous factors (such as the severity of the motor and communication deficits, and previous social behavior), many persons with aphasia attest to the importance of the presence of role models within the family. In contrast, they note with disappointment and occasional bitterness that friends and acquaintances often abandon them at a certain point. Mr. D. was quite troubled by this observation.

> "We are put aside. Things aren't the same anymore with my friends. I used to have many friends; I lost them all. It's not the same. I want to discuss, to explain something, but I can't any more." He adds, "Some people I know, I don't stop to talk to them, I just can't. What will I say to them? I can no longer talk about much."

In response to whether it is he who is abandoning his friends or vice versa, he states:

> "I went twice to visit friends. I noticed that it's no longer the same with them. Me, I'm no longer the same person, and them, they tell me that they're busy, they have to go. That can really hurt!"

Mrs. P. had a similar experience: "At first we are surrounded by people, but later they all withdraw."

A recent German study[5] in which the researchers interviewed over 20 brain-injured patients as well as their families, clearly revealed that the psychosocial repercussions of aphasia affect not only the person with aphasia, but also the family. The results of this investigation corroborate American studies[1,4] which suggest that persons with aphasia and their families inevitably experience *social restriction,* which is only indirectly related to the severity of the motor or language impairments resulting from aphasia. Instead, it stems from the *social stigmatization* that affects the family as a whole. The researchers thus describe them as "aphasic families." In this study, 65% of the families noticed a decline, in some cases even a total suspension, in their former social lives.

Up until the night before the fateful *event,* the person with aphasia was beforehand an integral part of society, considering himself a lifetime member, without ever questioning his status. He was society, along with his family, friends, colleagues, his barber, dentist, and to some extent everyone with whom he had ever dealt, even occasionally. Has the person with aphasia lost his place in this large social circle? Must he now be a mere onlooker to the daily activities of the *others* who are firmly *ensconced* within society? This new perspective soon leads the person with aphasia to closely examine the other contenders in this bout for life, where his own goal has become that of reinsertion while that of the others is to integrate him within their social network. Who are these opponents with whom he must interact?

THE PERSON WITH APHASIA IN SOCIETY

Apart from loved ones, the first members of society with whom persons with aphasia interact are health-care professionals. These specialists are some of the *others* who attempt to help and understand persons with aphasia. Are these health-care professionals invariably well-informed in their approach? Certainly they are aware (or have at least a theoretical knowledge) of the difference between aphasia and confusion or general intellectual deterioration. However, slowness, reduced memory, and attention span, perseveration, and comprehension difficulties that are frequently associated with aphasia sometimes generate some doubts in the minds of health-care professionals. What about the uneasiness sparked by the difficulties encountered in verbal communication? Should one speak in the person's place?

Some specialists react with exaggerated cordiality, and compensate for the person's *silence* by emitting a constant stream of conversation. Helen Wulf, a person with aphasia, recounts an anecdote in her book[8] about a therapist who spoke constantly while asking her to perform motor tasks. She describes the difficulty in discriminating and deciphering the instructions in the midst of the excessive discourse. The therapist would then point out poor concentration!

Helen Wulf brought up another thought-provoking experience: Professionals are aware of the isolation which threatens patients with aphasia, involuntarily or not, due to their communication difficulties. They therefore ensure that such a situation does not arise. During the patients' hospital stay, they attempt to promote maximal contact between the person with aphasia and other patients, during the hours that are not occupied by treatment. The author insists, however, that persons with aphasia could benefit from a certain degree of isolation, at least temporarily, that would enable them to relax and withdraw into an inner sanctum, cosy and warm, where there is no schedule to follow, and no effort required. This *retreat,* which everyone needs at some point, is unfortunately sometimes viewed as a negative behavior. Moreover, when patients with aphasia wish to practice on their own the exercises prescribed by the speech pathologist, they need tranquillity. They must withdraw to a setting which is far from the bustle of the corridor and the noise which filters into their rooms, to which they are more sensitive than ever. Helen Wulf had to constantly insist that the door to her room be closed, a request that worried certain health-care workers because it would subsequently be more difficult to watch her. They also feared that this behavior was a sign of isolation. Did they perhaps forget that the person with aphasia is, above all, an individual with **unique** psychosocial responses?

Mr. L., in an interview nine months after his stroke, recalled that at the beginning of his stay in a rehabilitation ward, he preferred not to receive visitors.

> "I asked everyone, even my wife, not to come to the hospital. I preferred being alone, I was much happier when people didn't come to see me. Once a week is quite enough. I couldn't speak. It would take me half an hour to talk, and by the end I would be drenched in sweat. It took a lot of will and energy."

He explained that although he was not depressed, his word-finding difficulties in conversations "put too much pressure" on him. Furthermore, he added that he cried on several occasions, which ultimately made him feel better; he did not wish to do so in the presence of friends or family.

A hyperemotional state often accompanies aphasia. Patients may burst into tears or even laughter or may utter strings of curses; all of which is beyond their control and under the circumstances is inappropriate. The fact that they are unable to express their regret or offer excuses contributes to the person's embarrassment in this situation. Rather than releasing tension, these manifestations may be themselves a source of shame not only for the person with aphasia, but also for the family. The family may ultimately shun social occasions, for fear that the person with aphasia will embarrass them, particularly when the slightest incident, inoffensive to others, triggers vulnerability and an outburst of emotion in the person with aphasia.

Once the first round (the acute phase that consumes all physical and mental energy) is won, persons with aphasia decide to fight on. They dare to take their first steps inside the circle and **reenter** society. They are immediately stunned by the intensity of the struggle and they strain against the indifference of the other players, themselves preoccupied by their own efforts to win this momentous game: the battle of everyday existence. The person with aphasia is an unexpected intruder. No one thought to reserve a place for him, **his place**. In fact, is it really him? He is not easily recognizable. Everyone is in a hurry, yet he is slow. How can he find a place on the team?

The Obstacle Course

Noise, movement, pushing, and shoving all heighten the person's insecurities. Due to difficulties with mobility and coordination compounded by slowed mental operations and impaired communication, persons with aphasia prefer to shun stimulating environments. If they do not live alone, and if the family displays comprehension rather than resignation, they will gradually readjust to society. For example, they can plan their schedules so as to avoid shopping and visiting businesses during peak periods. Persons with aphasia who live alone, however, will require more time to develop their own adaptation strategies; an alternative may be complete abandonment of a formerly routine social activity.

Transactions

The person with aphasia can no longer qualify for the speed competitions which are a hallmark of modern society. In fact, persons with aphasia can best cope with only *one thing at a time*. They are slow: Often they have the use of only one hand — not the most coordinated one! — to handle packages, wallets, and often their canes. They must concentrate to register and comprehend the amounts that cashiers spew at them, sometimes mumbled with their back to the person with aphasia, before they hurriedly move on to the next customer. In their endeavors to extract bills from their wallets, persons with aphasia most often neglect to verify if the amount is correct, partly because the calculation would take too long and partly because they can sense the impatience of the other customers in line. A young woman with aphasia stated:

> "I hate the cash at the grocery. People push. I put the money in my wallet (with) one hand, I don't have time to explain. Everyone is in a hurry, they push my things. I prefer to keep quiet."

In addition, many persons with aphasia often find it difficult to understand figures. Did the cashier say $12.45, $45, or $4.05? At the grocery store or at the bank, people with aphasia must ask the clerk to repeat several times, feeling guilty about wasting other people's time or automatically they confidently present a bill of large denomination and hope to receive the appropriate change.

> "At the bank, I hated dealing with the teller; she worked fast, but my mind works slower. She counted the money, I stopped counting it."

Society is always on the run. There is no room for slowness, hesitation, and inefficiency. Some are almost surprised that people with disabilities even dare to try to enter the rat race.

Restaurants

Eating at a restaurant is generally a pleasurable and even festive experience. Yet for some persons with aphasia, particularly those who have a low tolerance for noise, this is yet another social activity which they would rather avoid. In an attempt to please his wife, a person with aphasia, one spouse made reservations at her favorite restaurant. Unfortunately, he had neglected to mention that he wanted a table in a quiet section. He quickly requested a table change when his wife, blocking her ears, wanted to leave the restaurant. Another spouse of a person with aphasia who was in a rehabilitation program described to the speech pathologist how her husband was stared at in a restaurant because his partial facial paralysis prevented him from eating properly. Elaine, a young woman with aphasia, explained that even though she never gave up the habit of dining out regularly, at first she deliberately ordered foods which she could cut with one hand, with her fork. "I never stopped going out with normal people, but I just about died inside." A few years later, now that she gained more self-assurance, Elaine simply asks for her food to be cut in advance. She has noticed that people gladly comply with this request. She has come to realize: "We eat slowly, fast food is not for us."

Public Transport

Having few motor disabilities, Elaine is still able to take the subway, yet she feels limited by her communication problems. How can she request, understand, or offer information? "It is hard to speak. When people would ask me directions in the subway, I wished I could disappear! I signalled to them that I was unable to speak. I looked away. I thought to myself: *They think I am crazy, that I do not want to explain!* Once, when trying to give a woman directions, she stammered, and noticed the listener's puzzlement. "She hesitated, she didn't trust me." Elaine adds "I am scared of making mistakes." She is also disturbed by the jostling crowds in the subway system. When she must ask a stranger for directions: "People think I am Hispanic. I am scared that they will address me in Spanish." It often happens that people with aphasia acquire a kind of foreign accent that, in fact, stems from their articulatory difficulties. For them, this is a cause of considerable embarrassment because it further weakens their self-image; they have enough trouble defining their identity, torn between this new person who is disabled physically and socially and their previous personality which is still influential, and yearns for self-expression.

Mr. M., although he is distressed by his condition, has not lost his sense of humor. He related the following anecdote. After he explained to a taxi driver that he had communication problems, the driver, who had misunderstood, asked him if he was from a foreign country. Even after Mr. M. replied that he was not, the driver insisted: "Where are you from?" Mr. M., exasperated, quipped, "I come from Aphasia. Where is that? In the south of France!" Another woman recounts that a taxi driver refused to serve her because she could not clearly pronounce the address. He apparently thought she was drunk.

The Telephone

The telephone is the most dreaded enemy for most persons with aphasia. Many have experienced the horror of being treated as drunk or drugged due to their lack of intelligibility in telephone conversations. Most persons with aphasia flee from these dreaded exchanges, at least in the first few months after the onset of the condition, and sometimes even longer. For some, even dialling a number correctly is so demanding that they subsequently forget what they wanted to say, or to whom they wanted to speak, particularly when the call is an important one. If the listener becomes impatient with his word-finding difficulties, the person with aphasia panics and begins to stammer. Everyone has had the unpleasant experience of being passed from one person to another, and having to repeat the same message over and over. This procedure exasperates and drains the person with aphasia, ultimately leading to discouragement.

Calling a taxi, giving the right address, making or cancelling a dentist appointment, understanding the time of the appointment or explaining why that time is inconvenient, are all seemingly innocuous situations in daily life which can be extremely complicated for people with aphasia. They are forced to rely on others for many such details, or else bravely confront frustrating and sometimes humiliating situations.

In this era where society is racing ahead at breakneck speed, it is not surprising that people with aphasia tend to retreat into isolation. They have no alternative but to perceive themselves as outsiders. It is only with a great deal of determination and confidence in themselves, and — in spite of it all — in others, that people with aphasia can, in the best cases, eventually adapt by reaching compromise solutions and adopting compensatory strategies which help simplify their lives. What can society do to reduce the number of obstacles which persons with aphasia face in their daily lives? We must find means of smoothing their paths and facilitating their integration.

MUTUAL ADJUSTMENTS

To *persons with aphasia,* social reintegration involves better planning of outings, the setting of priorities in their activities, and learning to recognize what is feasible given their current limitations. They must also remain open to the exploration of other interests. All in all, people with aphasia must keep in mind that they are partly responsible for their reintegration in society. Clay Dahlberg[(2)], a doctor who acquired aphasia, agrees that patients must play active roles in their own recovery. They must proceed at their own pace and create a new way of life for themselves throughout each stage of recovery.

The role of *society* is to ease the reintegration of people with aphasia by manifesting a sincere desire to understand their experience in order to create a physical and social environment which will be most conducive for communication.

The first stage of this process is contingent upon society being well informed about aphasia and its associated symptoms. The next step is for society to reassess some of its current values. As we have seen, society favors autonomy, output, efficiency, and time-saving. How, therefore, can the person with aphasia find a place in society? Speed is the person's enemy.

Persons with Aphasia must Adapt

Persons must learn to live **with** their aphasia. The first step towards social reintegration is to **recognize** that they are *different,* this is the only way they will come to accept themselves as they are. Secondly, persons with aphasia must seek to overcome obstacles, to develop and adopt strategies which will allow them to function at their own pace, in the scope of their limitations and abilities. For example, to avoid misunderstandings, they can give the taxi driver a piece of paper on which they have written the address of their destination. Carrying identification on their person is compulsory. Persons with aphasia are no longer hesitant about presenting their aphasia association membership cards in order to inform people about their condition.

However, most persons with aphasia, virtually ashamed of their deficient verbal performance, prefer isolation. They flee social encounters rather than explain from the start that their language problem is a result of aphasia. Most people with aphasia take several months, even years, to recognize and accept the fact that aphasia is not necessarily well known, and that people are often unable to guess what type of disability they are facing with in the person with aphasia. Eventually, the person with aphasia comes to realize that impatience, intolerance, and even arrogance on the part of listeners will quickly give way to indulgence when they are informed that the speaker has the sequels of an illness rather than those of a mental disability or alcoholism.

We have already mentioned that telephone calls are the dread of many persons with aphasia. Numerous people with aphasia systematically avoid this mode of communication, yet others develop strategies for facilitating telephone use. Those who can, write in advance a few key words on a piece of paper. Others report that before calling, they practice aloud, especially when the call is important. Elaine admits that she spent some time just warning the caller about her language impairment.

> "I got very nervous speaking on the phone. People thought I was drunk, they would cut me off, then I got blocked. Now, I start off by saying I have aphasia. I say, *please, madam, would you kindly be patient so you can understand me?"*

Mr. L. learned early on to warn the listener of his speaking impairment: "If not, they would think that I'm senile or a child!" When he must give a phone number, he writes it out several times on a piece of paper, and then repeats it two or three times to the listener. He then asks the other person to read back the number while he checks it against what he wrote on the page. Mr. L. claims: "There's a trick to it. After a while you get the trick." Elaine concludes: "The first thing to do is to explain your situation. It's a morale booster. You feel awful, you explain yourself and at once you feel better."

Other dilemmas are ultimately resolved by other solutions. Persons with aphasia thus learn to reorganize their daily routine and to rethink their schedules. To avoid noise, crowds, and long waits in line, they now refrain from visiting banks, stores, or taking the subway during peak periods.

For people who formerly led active lives, it is hard to accept that confusion and frustration threaten them if they do more than one thing at a time. For some, performing a verbal and physical activity simultaneously can overload their powers of concentration, at least for those who also have significant motor disabilities. Most persons with aphasia are no longer able to read or even to speak if the television or radio is on.

Helen Wulf[8] reluctantly admitted that she could not perform physical exercises, although part of her daily routine, if she became distracted by other thoughts. She had to count along with the exercises, or else she would get lost. Her experience as a mother and an associate in her husband's business accustomed her to solving two or three simultaneous problems easily and quickly. It was frustrating for her to realize that she could no longer engage in more than one activity at a time. She was subsequently forced to structure her time and activities and take on help, e.g. hire a maid. Other people have found it difficult to relegate to their spouse or colleagues responsibilities in which they previously excelled. As Mr. L. explains:

> "Just the idea that I am unable to do anything disturbed me so much that it took me an hour and a half to calm down. I know that there are people who do things for me, and I know I can't do them any more; I would have liked to be able to do things on my own. But I learned not to strain myself."

In addition, **fatigue** is another obstacle which may arise at any time and with which the person with aphasia must learn to cope. Persons with aphasia must learn to identify the signs in order not to become exhausted and risk disaster, such as frustration and discouragement in the face of difficulties which suddenly seem impossible to overcome. Particularly at the onset of the illness, fatigue is an unremitting cloud hanging over the person's head. A simple and familiar activity lasting only a few minutes can provoke an overwhelming fatigue in the person with aphasia. It may be difficult for the family to understand this phenomenon, especially since the person with aphasia is often unable to convey this experience verbally. It is an important aspect to keep in mind: in some cases a therapy session may have to be cancelled, or a plan may have to be postponed. Of course, these adjustments demand the comprehension and cooperation of the person's family.

Society must also Adjust

While many persons with aphasia are still capable of verbal communication, their performance is no longer as smooth and spontaneous as before. Most often, verbal production is self-conscious and laborious because the words are not easily accessible. The process may be draining for persons with aphasia, especially because in order to express their message, they must be given ample time. If the persons feel rushed, they will stammer, get stuck, and even cease communicating all the ideas in their mind that are begging to be expressed. Helen Wulf[8] discussed the degree of great frustration that she felt because she had so many interesting things to say which were very clear in her mind. Unfortunately, she lacked the desired precision and nuances in her speech. For this reason, she stresses that in order to truly help persons with aphasia communicate, the listener must approach them calmly and take the time to listen to them with a sincere desire to learn what they want to say; one should especially avoid leaping to conclusions.

David Knox[6] recalls misunderstandings arising from his tendency to interpret literally his wife's imprecise or inexact aphasic utterances. With time, he learned that a person with aphasia may find it difficult to describe even mundane events; key words may be misused or absent. He subsequently learned not to reply immediately during a conversation, so that he could review the entire message, taking into account the situational context from which it arose.

It is essential to find a balance between speaking in the persons' stead when they cannot find the right words and end up leaving it to family members to complete the message, and anticipating the persons' utterances at the first sign of hesitation. Elaine claims: "It was tiring. I didn't look for words or try hard. I let my sister talk. I was afraid that people wouldn't understand." She adds, however, "People want to help you talk. It is worse. People find a word, it blocks my thoughts."

Obviously we should learn the subtle art of being active listeners!

Another frustrating situation for persons with aphasia is when they find themselves in the midst of a conversation without being truly integrated by the other speakers. It often happens that people speak exclusively to the person's companion, even to the point that they do not even glance at the person with aphasia. Moreover, trying to engage a conversation in an environment with the only noise being the buzz of nearby conversations magnifies his comprehension difficulties. The person is no longer able to filter the conversation from the surrounding noise. We can help people with aphasia escape from this din by taking them aside.

Finally, while psychosocial adjustment, as much for persons with aphasia as for their families, largely depends on the ability to accept and to integrate new roles, it also depends on the **indispensable** — but all too often inadequate — support from society in general, including health-care workers, community centers, associations for persons with aphasia or with other disabilities, municipal and governmental agencies, accessible buildings and transport, and subsidies for associations and dissemination of information about aphasia.

Time to Live

The TIME factor is constantly mentioned by people with aphasia. First of all, it takes them *time* to understand what is happening to them. We also know that it takes time for people with aphasia to express themselves. It is essential, therefore, that we also **take the time** to listen as well as to talk to them, without necessarily demanding an answer in return, especially at first. All they expect from us is a warm greeting, to be recognized as people in fine mental health, and to be shown understanding, patience, and indulgence. They wish for a smile and a human contact. In addition, they should be encouraged to persevere with their efforts and they should be reminded that rehabilitation also takes **time**!

A man in his 30s, an insurance representative before he acquired aphasia, reports that a year and a half after the onset of his illness: "It's hard, but life is wonderful! I had always forgotten to *take the time to live.* Now, it feels good, taking my time. I even meet new friends when I go for my treatments."

Elaine, a woman in her forties, with aphasia for 11 years, would like to tell other persons with aphasia not to avoid social relations for too long: "Oh, go for it!" she suggests with conviction. She adds:

> "Friendly advice: Live from day to day. Time settles lots of things. Now I appreciate each moment, each minute. Before always hurrying, fast, fast. I appreciate nature, walking in the forest; it's nice, it's calm, (I) take the time to listen to the birds, which bothered me before."

Of course, the change in lifestyle is rather radical. Yet although the world of the person with aphasia may be shrunk by circumstance, psychologist Colette Durieu[3] insists that "a shrunken world, if it remains open, will sustain the desire to live." With the help of their families, people with aphasia can learn that not all pleasures in life are language bound!

When team members do not get along well, adjustments become absolutely necessary. Learning to get acquainted, taking individuals into account, making sure the *rules* are flexible, accepting changes in habits, for the person with aphasia as well as for society, in other words, adjusting to limitations on time, space, noise, communication, under new and different conditions are all strategies that can lead to victory: A **successful reintegration** of the person with aphasia into society.

REFERENCES

1. Artes, R.& R. Hoops: Problems of aphasic stroke patients as identified by patients' wives, **in** *Recovery in Aphasics,* Lebrun, Y. & R. Hoops (eds.), Swets and Zeitlinger, Amsterdam, 1976.

2. Dahlberg, C.C. & J. Jaffe: *Stroke. A doctor's personal story of his recovery,* W.W. Norton and Company Inc., New York, 1977.
3. Durieu, C.: *La rééducation des aphasiques,* Psychologie et Sciences Humaines, Charles Dessart (ed.), Brussels, 1969.
4. Feibel, J.H. & C.J. Springer: Depression and failure to resume social activities after stroke. *Arch Phys Med Rehabil,* **63,** 1982.
5. Herrmann, M. & C.W. Wallesh: Psychological changes and psychosocial adjustment with chronic and severe non-fluent aphasia. *Aphasiology,* **2,** 1989.
6. Knox, D.: *Portrait of Aphasia,* Wayne State University Press, Detroit, 1971.
7. Schmidt & Coll.: Status of Stroke Patients: A Community Assessment. *Arch Phys Med Rehabil,* **67(Feb)**, 1986.
8. Wulf, H.: *Aphasia, my world alone,* Wayne State University Press, Detroit, 1973.

CHAPTER 13

THE PERSON WITH APHASIA AND THE WORKFORCE

J. ROLLAND AND C. BELIN

INTRODUCTION

What happens when patients with aphasia no longer require the services of health-care facilities such as hospitals or rehabilitation centers which had taken care of them up until then? Such persons *still* face numerous problems. Below we will devote particular attention to the topic of persons with aphasia in the workforce.

The presence of aphasia has often been considered a negative factor for brain-injured patients who wished to return to work. Weisbroth, Esibil, and Zuger[8] demonstrate that among subjects with right hemiplegia the presence of a major communication impairment is a statistically significant factor which divides patients into two sub-groups: Those who do and those who do not return to work. In the same vein, Howard et al.[5] revealed that, of patients who return to work, twice as many have lesions in the right hemisphere than in the left. In contrast, Oder et al. profess that for patients with motor disabilities, the severity of the aphasia has no long-term effect on the prognosis.

Most of the studies cite the percentage of patients who return to work: 36% of the 600 persons with aphasia studied by Ducarne de Ribaucourt[3]; a mere 20% of the patients with *severe* chronic aphasia examined by Herrmann and Wallesch[4] were capable of adequately performing household chores. These two examples are proof of the variability that can be obtained from this type of questionnaire. In fact it is impossible to dissociate the return to work from many other factors, of which the severity of aphasia rather than the actual type of aphasia may be the key element[7].

There is no standardized means of assessing residual capacities which indicate a possible return to work. Therapists must therefore independently establish vocational evaluation programs, taking into account various elements of the patient's particular context. Naturally, this assessment is difficult, and must take many factors into consideration (e.g. age, motor and sensory disabilities, psychological problems, medical history, the patient's motivation, as well as the employer's attitude). Overall, each patient should be perceived as an individual, and each case should be considered separately. The patient's family also plays a major role: Some patients are overprotected, while others are left to fend for themselves.

Social factors also commonly influence whether or not a person with aphasia can eventually return to work.

- Social security policies are most often based on the 'all or nothing' principle: Complete reintegration or total disability. There is generally a great deal of red tape to wade through in order to qualify for part-time employment.

- Certain patients prefer the security of a disability pension to the risk of failure at the workplace.

In Brussels, Belgium, there is a program, developed by Xavier Seron, in which people can participate in a pre-professional job placement outside of the Rehabilitation Center. The program lasts six months, during which the patient, the employer, and the therapist work together to develop a gradual reintegration in the workforce. The schedule, pace, and the type of work are adapted to the patient's residual disabilities. To our knowledge, the Belgian system has no counterpart in any other francophone European nation.

COTOREP is a French organization that serves disabled persons. Its goal is the social and professional reintegration of its clients. Yet few persons with aphasia actually find practical assistance there; none of the people who were contacted during our survey were able to procure employment through this organization.

In order to determine as clearly as possible the chief problems which persons with aphasia face in their return to work, we have undertaken the following study. Our goals were to identify the difficulties which surface during job searches, during professional reintegration, as well as when a return to work is impossible. The cases of six typical patients were selected, to serve as illustrations, from a general survey population. The six patients are young, with moderate aphasia which still allows for adequate communication, moderate to no motor disabilities, and living in socio-economic conditions and family environments that reduce the likelihood of other social problems. Thus they are free to choose whether or not to return to work.

The responses below were given by persons with post-stroke aphasia. Note that patients with head trauma generally present severe diffuse symptoms; subsequently, their experience is not identical to that of stroke patients. In cases where aphasia is induced by a tumor — a generally irreversible condition over a varying period of time — patients are not likely to encounter problems with professional reintegration.

THE SURVEY

Sixty-three patients were studied in this survey. Of these, 6 belong to socio-cultural level 3: i.e. at least 14 years of school education. These patients are between 23 and 54 years of age. Thirty-two belong to socio-cultural level 2: 10 to 12 years of school; they are 32 to 51 years old. Finally, 25 belong to socio-cultural level 1: 6 to 8 years of school; they are 35 to 53 years old.

All subjects completed detailed questionnaires, and patients who reported prototypical difficulties were called in for an interview. The most revealing characteristics of their problems were duly noted.

According to the study, it appears that:

- it is extremely rare that patients return to a job that is equal to the one they previously held; no such cases were recorded in this study;
- some businesses (banks, for example) will sometimes offer modified jobs (reduced hours, less demanding tasks), but these arrangements are exceptional, and reflect the goodwill of the employer or the personnel manager;
- those who found jobs did so thanks to their own efforts;
- the family plays an essential role in this process.

The study reveals that when patients are overprotected and considered as highly diminished (even when their symptoms are moderate), no efforts are made to help them. The family neither helped nor encouraged the person to return to work. In these cases, it is very rare for patients to reintegrate into a profession, even though they may be motivated to do so. In the inverse scenario, where families are optimistic and enthusiastic, they can contribute greatly to the person's ability to muster and sustain the motivation essential for a return to work.

Below are the cases of six typical patients with aphasia; four of these patients returned to work, two remained unemployed.

Of the four patients who found jobs:

The *first* subject is a student (CL3: 14 years of education), 23, who returned to school at a lower level.

The *second* case is that of a secretary (CL2: 10 years of education) a 34-year-old mother who resumed part-time work in the home.

The *third* case is that of a businessman (CL2: 12 years of education) 51, who found work in the Val de Loire Aphasia Association.

The *fourth* case is that of a commercial farmer (CL1: 7 years of education), 49, who resumed work on the farm *at his own pace.*

These subjects all enjoyed fine motor recovery, and their language disabilities were minor. Furthermore, all benefited from support from their family.

The two cases where subjects did not return to work consist of the following:

The *first* is a teacher, 38, who could not reintegrate into her former profession despite her initiative. Her field demanded a level of recovery of both motor and language abilities which she was unable to attain.

The *second* case involves a businesswoman, 40, who ran a beauty salon. Her return to professional activities was particularly hampered by her residual motor disabilities, as well as by a lack of motivation, and an unsupportive family.

In spite of the difficulties the two subjects faced, in the former case there was significant motivation to resume work, while this was lacking in the latter case. Nonetheless, both subjects in these examples were unable to procure employment.

Common symptoms found in both patients include severe disabilities linked to residual right hemiplegia (they could, however, walk unaided), insufficient language skills to communicate adequately (e.g. they experienced word-finding difficulties, generally semantic paraphasias, reduced verbal fluency, and dysarthria); finally, in both cases the patient's family was clearly averse to the person's professional reintegration.

THE PATIENTS' RESPONSES

F.R., female, 38, a teacher, ambidextrous.
Etiology: stroke, aneurism in the left frontal region.
Motor disabilities: right hemiplegia.
Clinical type of aphasia: Broca's aphasia.

Before the illness, Ms. R. taught history and geography. She never completely recovered her motor skills: Her right arm is functionally disabled; she is capable of walking unassisted, although she does so with difficulty. The symptoms of aphasia have abated considerably. The effects are currently very moderate, and are limited to dysarthria, more acute late in the day and when the patient tires, along with word-finding difficulties and reduced verbal fluency.

F.R. began reintegration three years after the onset of the illness:

> "I wanted to pursue a master's degree in medieval history, that really fascinated me, but physically and practically . . . *I had no choice but to quit,* anyways, I applied myself for three months. That was really absolutely too tiring. But later, when my children will be a bit older, I will try again. My husband insisted that I stop. He would say: *Later, we shall see.*
>
> "So I thought I could work as a librarian, but they informed me that there were no jobs, that it would be difficult . . . I wanted to use this vocation as a means of having access to medieval archives, but I was not able to do so. No one wanted to listen to me, nor to try to understand. The principals that I spoke to did not take my problems very seriously. You see, what happens to others doesn't count for much. People are rather selfish, they don't make an effort to try to solve your problems, or even get involved to a certain extent.

"I wanted to try to resume my former occupation, but I was refused . . . because I was an auxiliary not a permanent teacher. I couldn't even find work as a substitute. What is more, *they considered me to be physically unfit.* I tire easily, that's true, but still, I'm quite hardy. That, however, is hard to prove.

"People suggested that perhaps I could find work supervising students in study hall. That I could not accept, not after having worked as a teacher. Even then they said *maybe.*

"I was interviewed by someone at the Education Office regarding a possible return to teaching, but the person informed me that the work would be too physically and emotionally demanding. I did not insist (what would that have accomplished?) because I used to have a good deal of authority. Although I was strict, my students were quite fond of me. I always thought that if my mind goes blank, the students will act up, and that's something I never want to happen. Just imagine, as I entered the class, the students would burst out laughing because I hobble.

"I also know that to this day *I tire much more easily and I am much slower.* I also get the impression that when I do not say something . . . if I want to keep it to myself, to say it later, I forget it. It's really awful, I interrupt conversations... because of this problem. It's also true that if I don't pay attention, if I don't concentrate enough, I will forget to do things . . . *I tend to be more scatterbrained now. All these factors make it quite difficult to return to work, especially to a job like mine.* Yet I refuse to give up, I tell myself that I will try again in two years when my son will be in elementary school. Then, I will start over.

"My husband, however, feels that I should stay home, he thinks I am just asking for aggravation and fatigue. He accepts that I return to work as long as I don't tire myself out, you know, it's impossible . . . You always get somewhat tired when you work."

Ms. R. was dissuaded by the Education Office in her attempts to resume her former teaching position. Neither could she secure a job as a substitute teacher. Her efforts to find work as a librarian were unsuccessful, while her husband, fearing that she would overexert herself, was also averse to her return to work.

In this case we can observe the usual problems that impede a return to work: Fatigue, slowness, reduced attention span, forgetfulness, along with residual motor difficulties, and the consequences of aphasia. The patient suffers as well due to employers' lack of comprehension, and family members' negative views regarding her return to work.

Ms. R. is aware of her difficulties but is still hopeful that she can pursue her profession and even advanced studies (i.e., a master's in history) in the near future.

This case exemplifies an apparent paradox whereby the will to believe in potential success in the future is coupled with awareness of the difficulties arising from a disability as well as other problems which originate from a workforce which is closed or hostile to the person's reentry.

The patient above overestimates her abilities and remains optimistic for the future despite the presence of concrete hurdles. She typifies a certain category of persons with aphasia which we considered worthy of discussion.

J.T., female, 40, right-handed, businesswoman.
Etiology: stroke, infarct in the left thalamus.
Motor disabilities: right hemiplegia.
Clinical type of aphasia: severe thalamic aphasia.

Before the illness, J.T. operated a beauty salon. She has not completely recovered her motor abilities; her right arm is still weak. The patient has difficulties walking, though she can walk without assistance. J.T. underwent speech therapy for two years. She is currently experiencing dysarthria, reduced verbal fluency, and a diminished capacity to produce complex utterances. The patient still experiences memory lapses; however, they are less severe than at the onset of the illness.

J. T. did not resume her former occupation. Given the motor disabilities, it was unrealistic to consider working in the same profession. It would have been possible, however, for the patient to hire a manager and thus participate indirectly in the operation of the business. This was exactly what Mrs. T. had in mind early in her convalescence,

> "But I didn't fully realize . . . still, my husband tried to make it clear to me that I would find it very hard . . .
>
> "I didn't go back to my old job, it was impossible. I didn't have any other professional skills, so starting over somewhere else . . . was out of the question. *I did feel, however, that I was capable of doing clerical work, filing, preparing documents, mailing.* I called someone about a job as a librarian's aide, and I made it clear that I tired easily, and that I worked slowly. They told me *not to even think about it.* So I didn't insist any more. And my husband would always say to me: *Don't go all out, you'll never make it.* I must say that my husband did not want me to work again. I think he was right . . . He thought it was quite enough if I kept busy looking after our two children and taking care of the

housework. It's true, it took me quite some time before I became at all efficient, and even then I'm not quick; I simply don't do the same work, I always need to ask for help, I just don't have the same energy level. What still bothers me is my faulty memory. It is better than before, but I still have problems. I forget all kinds of things, but I got into the habit of writing everything down. So for at least two years now, I take care of the children when they come home from school, I feed them, I make them do their homework and recite their lessons. When things start to get out of hand, my husband will help when he gets home. Even now, now that my recovery is . . . complete . . . better than we hoped, I don't think I will return to work. I think my husband is right. I tire easily, I forget things, I take everything very slowly, so there is really no way I can work outside the home."

Evidently, in this case, the motor and neuropsychological disabilities significantly hamper the patient's professional reintegration. Moreover, the influence of the family clearly sways the patient away from the working world.

J.G. male, 22, right-handed, student.
Etiology: stroke, left rolandic angioma.
Motor disabilities: right hemiplegia.
Clinical type of aphasia: Broca's aphasia.
Associated disabilities: decreased sensitivity.

J.G. was a second-year student in an X-ray technician training program when he first experienced symptoms. On September 17, 1986, he underwent an operation for an angioma in the left rolandic region. The repercussions were grave: Right hemiplegia and severe language impairment, initial mutism as well as Broca's aphasia. Speech therapy was initiated at the earliest opportunity, along with physical therapy. The patient recovered fairly quickly; one year later he considered returning to school.

At that time, J.T. still had aphasia-related problems such as relatively mild dysarthria and word-finding difficulties:

"I audited a Red Cross course at the end of the school year. That didn't work out at all. I was having a hard time following. I wasn't able to understand everything. It was too fast, and I would lose track of what the teacher was saying. I got tired very easily. But I just went to this course so I could get my brain in shape. I had forgotten a lot, I thought *I have got to make an effort.*

"I wasn't able to continue on to third year, so, with the approval of the director of the Red Cross, I started second year again.

Before long it was obvious that I wasn't recovering the use of my right hand fast enough, so I had to quit. I learned to write with my left hand, but I wasn't adept enough . . . quick enough . . . I tried to adapt the right-hand movements to my left hand. They told me *take all the time you need'.* Actually, *those were just empty words, because there was no concrete way that people helped me. None of the teachers cared about me, gave me one bit of advice or tried to make my disability less . . . unbearable.* What's more, a friend who worked for the Red Cross, a "physio," told me that the teachers wanted me to start over from scratch, from day one. So that, I just couldn't believe. They thought I just could not make it, but at the same time *there was a hell of a difference between their 'encouraging' words and the actual effects, which were nonexistent.*

"Also, there were training periods where we were responsible for five or six patients. The supervisor said . . . well, saw that I wasn't able to handle these patients because of my motor limitations.

"Of course, nobody made an effort to help me compensate for this problem, to teach me how to handle patients. Maybe there was a better way to function, but that . . . I'll never know.

"So at that point I decided to look for other opportunities.

"I decided to register with the Tours Chamber of Commerce. I was well received there. To be chosen, you must pass a few tests and an interview; they are not overly demanding. There, the training is no barrier for persons with physical disabilities. I write with my left hand, things go by a bit quickly for me, but it's not impossible. *At any rate, I am slower than before in just about everything. Luckily, these classes are easier, because my memory is not as strong, that's for sure. I have trouble concentrating. I also find it quite tough learning things by heart.* But I do have the motivation to make a huge effort, which I didn't have any more at the Red Cross. The effects of my disability are no longer the same, and, in this new vocation, I hope that I will be able to get by.

"When you graduate from here you can work as a wholesaler, 'goodsseller', [sic] a general salesman. If I can go further, I would like to work in commercial engineering. For the time being, I don't think about it . . . obviously.

"To sum it all up, I was lucky, because I was able to do something else. *Not because I received outside help, but thanks to my family, everyone at home who helped me stay confident so that I could seek knowledge that would never be mine if I didn't go out and get it. You've got to be active, you know, to succeed, and no one can do that on their own."*

It is obvious in this case that the patient's reintegration is a product of his and his family's combined efforts, and that no external help of any kind was offered.

Y.L., male, 51, right-handed (ambidextrous tendencies), businessman.
Etiology: stroke, aneurism in the left sylvian region.
Motor disabilities: right hemiplegia.
Clinical type of aphasia: Broca's.

Before the illness, Y.L. was a salesman. He underwent five and a half years of speech and physical therapy. Recovery of motor skills is complete: The effects of aphasia are limited to extremely moderate dysarthria, mild word-finding difficulties, a greater reduction in verbal fluency, and slow conceptualization.

Y.L. did not return to his former occupation. *Despite a successful recovery,* he felt diminished; his self-confidence was extremely low, he considered himself a burden on his family. He represents the category of person with aphasia which brand themselves *as severely disabled and marginalized for life, despite having only very mild symptoms.*

"I felt worthless, but it's true I did recover well. Later, when I believed that I might be good for something, I no longer thought about killing myself.

"But of course it was impossible for me to return to my old job. And yet I thought that I would be able . . . only . . . to do that, nothing else. But I realized there would be problems in working like I used to, that is to say travelling 300-500 km a day, placing orders, it was impossible. *It would take me too long.* Even talking to clients, I couldn't . . . I would get a headache after speaking to people for an hour.

"Also, you know, I used to speak two languages, now I can't even speak French. Reading and writing . . . no . . . it's too tough . . . when I read the newspaper, an hour later my head hurts. *And I can't speak like before,* I don't always say what I want. I also can't write a text. I need help. *I tire easily when I read,* or write, talk, or, well anything . . . *I have to stop often,* when I do something. I get tired very quickly.

"So now I work at the Val de Loire Aphasia Association. But I still have the same problems: *I have to work slowly,* and not for too long. I push myself to do more and more . . . but anyway, my productivity is still low.

"And *I have memory lapses,* I have to write everything down. The only reason I can work again is I work at my own pace, *my slowness* is not a limitation in my work. I only work around ten hours a week. By chance, I met people who I could work with, and we started this association. From then on, many things have changed for me.

"Before, I was earning money, now I take the time to live. And I try to help others. I meet people who are more disabled than I, and that stops me from complaining about my problems. I discovered another lifestyle and another way of seeing others. *Things in life don't have the same importance, not at all.*

"My social reintegration is fine. I feel comfortable in this association, I can help others in certain ways, but *as far as my professional reintegration, zero.* I'm telling you that *another job, even at a lower level, wouldn't be possible.*

"There is the problem of profitability, *no employer is pleased with a slow worker,* someone who tires quickly; you know, there is nothing set up with us in mind. We *have to deal with people who are more or less tolerant,* that's all, but their help doesn't go far. There are no set plans, *no laws to solve our problems.*

"I receive disability benefits. It is not my own doing, Social Security decided. They don't think I am able to . . . work. They think that I can't work at all. Even at odd jobs. We are considered useless, that's all. So we have to look on our own, make connections, ask friends, people around us, and sometimes it works. What I mean by 'it works' is *that we find an occupation rather than a real job.* But for me, things are finally working out. My life has direction once again. I am never bored."

Y.L.'s illness took a severe psychological toll. He went through a depressive period, and it took him some time to learn to enjoy life again. He seems to overestimate his residual disabilities, and his lack of confidence is still prominent. Despite a nearly complete recovery, this person who *formerly* had aphasia still feels quite diminished, incapable of performing the tasks which are a normal part of daily life. He constantly claims "I am no longer the same." Even so, with the help of family and friends, he mustered the will to find an occupation where he wholeheartedly applies himself in spite of the fact that he is in perpetual distress. Note that this an interesting scenario as it is commonly seen in cases of persons with aphasia.

M.-C. R., female, 34, right-handed, secretary.
Etiology: stroke, left sylvian aneurism.
Motor disabilities: right hemiplegia.
Clinical type of aphasia: amnesic aphasia, reduced language abilities.

Ms. R. was a former secretary, as well as an assistant dental technician. Mother of three children, she was pregnant when she underwent neurosurgery for a ruptured aneurism in the left sylvian region.

She had planned to return to work approximately one year after the onset of the illness. At that time, her language problems had nearly disappeared, the only disturbance was lingering word-finding difficulties. Her right hemiplegia had also abated significantly, and was subsequently apparent only in a slight decrease in muscular strength. She was particularly conscious of this disability when it came to caring for her baby. *She was unable to return to her former occupation.*

> "I still had difficulty talking, *I got very tired very quickly.* I thought that I could continue my work as assistant technician because that job is . . . well it's not with others, that is, you don't have to talk much; it's laboratory work. There is no . . . exchange . . . contact with the public, but I still tired far too easily, and the employer who I spoke to strongly discouraged me from working, even, apparently, on a part-time basis. I also noticed that *I was far slower,* my efficiency at home was not at all like before. My husband did not really encourage me to work outside the home. And I couldn't . . . you know . . . remem . . . concentrate like before. I often would forget things, people said that I was acting strange. Well, not strange, but dazed, and even now, I have to pay strict attention because my memory lapses are more . . . often . . . more common than before."

Two years later, M.-C. R. again attempted to reintegrate into her former profession. She contacted several dental surgeons and technicians.

There was a clear distinction between encouraging words and concrete help, that is to say actual job offers. "I would often hear *You'll find something, we can't hire you, but if you persevere, you will find a job. I would be surprised if you didn't, because your current problems are really minor.'"*

At no time did employers consider adapting a job to the patient's residual disability, for example by modifying schedules or offering part-time employment. It was by *chance* that the patient found a new job.

> "I agreed to hold a STANHOME[1] meeting in my home. The person who performed the demonstration knew that I wanted to return to work and said I could work for the company. She brought me to see the manager of STANHOME, who asked me to start . . . no . . . try out. The test was fine, ok, alright; in short, they told me I did well enough. I had to learn about the products,

[1] Company that sells household products in the home.

and be able to do . . . no . . . to present them at gatherings in people's homes, to homemakers who would want to use them. I had to write everything down on paper, each time, I was scared my memory would fail me . . . would play tricks on me . . . anyways it was need . . . necessary for me to write everything down. I wrote all about the products, their names, their uses, and the orders and list of things for each person. It's not easy . . . not simple at all. I even made mistakes several times. But in the end the results . . . the consequences were not serious . . . luckily for me.

"I was able to work at this job for the sole reason that it doesn't take up too much of my time, and that I can work when I want. I only hold three meetings per week. I don't work during the school vacation so it's better for my children and myself. Like this I have calm moments, and I get by.

"The problem that I have these days is that I am *slower and I tire more easily than before,* I am less patient, I get irritated quicker, and my husband says that now I'm aggressive. Me, I don't believe him; before I was younger, I . . . how . . . I wanted everything, I . . . I accepted everything, I was stupid. Now, no. I speak my mind."

In the case above, the patient recovered very well, yet she is still troubled by slowness, fatigue, and the inability to concentrate. In the workplace in particular, these are characteristics which are not conducive to optimal profitability and efficiency.

The employers, in this case dental surgeons and technicians, were indeed aware of these limitations. They were reticent about hiring persons with aphasia, such as M.-C. R., even though the language problem, a minor one, does not necessarily affect the job, which in this case did not involve interaction with the clients.

No compromises were proposed to M.-C. R., in view of her specific symptoms of aphasia. There were no concrete offers resulting from her job search. As she attests, it was *fortuitous* circumstances that landed her a job. That is, a chance encounter that she used to her advantage; her sincere desire to work and her motivation guided her to her current situation.

R.B., male, 49, right-handed, commercial farmer.
Etiology: stroke, left capsuloventricular hematoma.
Motor disabilities: right hemiplegia.
Clinical type of aphasia: Broca's aphasia.

Before his illness, R.B. was a commercial farmer. The motor recovery was somewhat complete, with a residual decrease of strength in the patient's right arm. R.B. underwent language and physical therapy at a rehabilitation center for a year and a half. His current disabilities are moderate: Word-finding difficulties, reduced verbal fluency, poorly elaborated speech, and intermittent phonemic paraphasias that sometimes appear during spontaneous language. Moreover, the patient's family and R.B. himself have complained of a memory loss which hampers the performance of everyday activities. There are also problems with calculation. It is therefore impractical that R.B. retain the accounting duties for his farm. The family no longer considers him to be dependable and reliable enough to be entrusted with important matters.

Nonetheless, the patient partially resumed his occupation. He is able to drive his tractor and can perform various light tasks.

"I am no longer good for much, but I can still help my wife and son. What's *tebi* . . . *teli* . . . terrible is that I tire so very very soon. I can do a bit, but not too . . . well, not enough . . . not much. It's true that I can drive the *bractor* (tractor) but soon *it's enough,* a few circuits, some moves . . . uh . . . *mareuvres* . . . maneuvers, and I'm beat.

"I feed the livestock. Helping out with the kowing (sowing) is ok, but I stop before the others. My wife says that my mind is gone, it's true . . . They have to *rerind* me all the time . . . of things to do, or me, nothing, or . . . not too much. I just can't remember, that's really something.

"I'm still lucky, before I could not write, or read well. Now, I more or less *recovered,* it'll be alright."

R. B.'s family claims that he has become quite emotional, and that his work is irregular. Sometimes he is able to persist in an activity, sometimes not; and he quickly gives up. As a result, his productivity is highly variable. His wife reports that if he is not asked to do a specific task, he will do nothing.

"He does everything slower. And you often have to repeat things, he does not always understand right away. He doesn't always express himself the way he wants to, and sometimes that aggravates him . . . but that, still, it's ok because we understand him just the same. He's made a lot of progress.

"He used to have ideas about what to plant. We don't grow the same thing every year, in the same place — it's better for the soil that way. You have to rotate the crops. Now it's my son that makes the decisions. We have 92 hectares, it's not nothing, you know . . . Anyway, we mustn't complain too much. He's come a long way, and we know that he's made a lot of progress, and anyway, as we said, he still participates in certain activities. But it won't be like before, that's for sure. Our son is thinking of leaving . . . He wants to work in town. I don't know what I'm going to do. I'll have to hire a farm laborer. But to do that I'd have to be sure that we'd have a good year."

Apparently, R.B. was able to partially return to work, since he is the owner of his farming operation. His family knows how to best harness his residual abilities. The difficulties reported include slowness, lack of initiative, memory lapses, and problems with calculation, which all considerably diminish the quality of his work output. Note that the language problems have not been singled out as the chief disability; the reason being R.B.'s profession does not place much emphasis on unimpaired oral communication.

SUMMARY

From the prototypical cases described above the following conclusions can be drawn.

In Cases where the Person did not Return to Work

The *first case* clearly illustrates that motivation alone is not sufficient to overcome obstacles, and that people who formerly held advanced positions have greater difficulties returning to work: There is a considerable gap between the status *before* the illness and that *after* the illness. A new job, even at a clearly inferior level, is often impossible to obtain.

In some cases patients possess a great degree of motivation to seek employment despite opposition from reticent or discouraging employers, and despite the misgivings of family members. Ultimately, the persons' residual disabilities force them to give up. F.R.'s case clearly exemplifies this situation.

The *second example* typifies patients who are not motivated to return to work, who are easily convinced by the family not to pursue outside activities, and who quickly succumb to the negative attitudes of employers. J.T.'s case illustrates such a scenario: She had a motor limitation that did not allow her to resume her former occupation. Nonetheless, she wished to be *partially* involved in the *operation* of her business (a beauty salon). She was quite easily discouraged by her husband. Later, refusal from a single employer, contacted about another job, was sufficient to squelch any further attempts to find employment.

Persons who Returned to Work

Note that *in the 4 cases,* all the persons retained a certain degree of motivation in their search for a new job, due to support from family members. With their family's help, they benefited from prime opportunities to go back to work, which they all seized. Independently, they discovered the means to obtain employment tailored to their motivation as well as their disabilities. In every case, the work schedule was reduced.

Common and persistent complaints from those who work are the following: Fatigue, short attention span, and poor memory (frequent lapses, *everything* must be written down . . . if possible), slowness of mental operations and in the performance of routine tasks, and oral communication difficulties (a consequence of the aphasia) which interfere particularly with professional and telephone conversations.

Boehringer[1] attempted to define the necessary conditions for a job which would be satisfactory for such patients, especially for employers, because it is these factors which will have the greatest influence on the patients' success and how long they are able to remain at the workplace. To Boehringer, **output** is the main criterion which should be considered the driving force in society. The author subsequently specifies various elements which will affect a person's productivity: Intrinsic and extrinsic skills, training, motivation, fatigue, and social adaptation.

The complaints gathered here can be summarized in terms of the elements specified above.

- **Fatigue** is the primary factor given by the patients to account for their difficulties, even their failure to integrate back into the workforce. Clearly persons with aphasia, and brain-injured patients in general, are overly susceptible to fatigue. They are therefore less efficient and have a considerably diminished attention span, leading to an increase in errors. Therefore, they require a less demanding work schedule that would be suitable for their condition. This is rarely proposed to persons with aphasia, and has an even smaller chance of feasibility. M.-C. R. illustrates this point by the fact that she found a made-to-measure job where she can work at her own pace.

- **Intrinsic skills** correspond to the patients' residual capacities which may be determined by a thorough neuro–psychological examination. These skills are often the initial limitations in the job search. An infinite amount of motivation cannot compensate for these disabilities.

- **Extrinsic skills** are those related to a given job (technical and specialized knowledge), along with concrete skills (such as the ability to use a telephone), which may be particularly troubling for a person with aphasia.

- **Training,** for Boehringer, is indispensable to lead the patients back to their former jobs, or enable them to adapt to a new occupation. This training is rarely proposed to persons with aphasia. Rather it is the patients themselves, (with the help of their families) who try to return to their former job or to find a new one. No concrete modifications are envisioned for job–seekers with aphasia. At times employers may demonstrate goodwill, but most are reluctant.

- **Motivation** is an extremely important factor. It arises partly from the pleasure that one can derive from successfully performing a given task, and partly from the social consequences of the job: The remuneration and social status. Unfortunately, these motivational factors are often negative, in nature reflecting the patient's insecurities, employers' prejudices, the fear of losing the job, and other aspects linked to society. As a result, some patients prefer the security of a disability pension to the hazards of the workplace, where they are confronted with endless difficulties.

• **Social adaptation** takes into account the problem of work schedules and interpersonal relations (hierarchical and nonhierarchical) within a work team.

Another feature common to all these patients is **character** and **personality changes.** These changes should also be considered a substantial disability that often impedes a return to work.

The cases below represent varying degrees of personality disturbances.

• J.T., for example, became rather indifferent. She lost all her fighting spirit, and is now malleable and passive.

• F.R., on the contrary, struggles, takes initiative, and demonstrates an astounding degree of optimism. She represents a paradox between an awareness of residual problems that are so severe that she cannot return to her former profession, and an overestimation of her current abilities which lead her to envision projects that are not fully feasible.

• Y.L. typifies patients who exhibit an enduring and irreversible lack of self confidence. Among the cases presented above, he was the patient who recovered best; yet at the same time, his psychological limitations are the most severe. He underestimates his abilities, and his job clearly does not reflect his true capacities. He is thus a classic example of the syndrome: *L'aphasie n'est plus, mais l'aphasique demeure* (Y. Joanette) (the aphasia disappears, but the person with aphasia remains).

• J.-C. G. is young, confident, and has successfully adapted to a new academic milieu. He has become less critical and had lowered his expectations so they are more modest. He expresses no regret about what he *might* have achieved previously. He even feels that his new direction is better than his former vocation.

• M.-C. R., like many young patients with aphasia, considers the family, rather than her residual disabilities, as justification for working at an undemanding job that does not require too much of her time and energy. She has become particularly cautious in her new lifestyle. She lacks self assurance, and hides this lack of self confidence by an aggressiveness that family members never observed before.

• R.B. has become indifferent. Although he wishes to work on his farm, he cares little about the results of his labor. He is passive, follows others. Without encouragement from family members to work, he reduces his activity to a minimum. He is oblivious to the consequences of his irregular work output.

Before concluding this chapter, we feel it is important to emphasize the courage of these patients who, quite often, despite the support from the immediate family, live in rather dramatic solitude. They feel they are alone in accepting their disability and a new self image, alone in confronting *others*, and alone in their quest for a new philosophy of life. Most persons with aphasia keep their chin up, leading those who observe them to be inspired by their courage. Persons who do not have aphasia often benefit by reacting with a sense of humility and moderation and a better perspective on their own life problems.

REFERENCES

1. Boehringer, C.: Rendement et séquelles neuropsychologiques: la remise au travail du patient cérébro-lésé, **in** *Rééduquer le cerveau: logopédie, psychologie, neurologie.* Seron, X. & C. Laterre (eds.), Pierre Mardaga, Brussels, 1982.
2. Coyette, F.: Neuropsychologie et ergothérapie. Réinsertion vie sociale et professionnelle. Texte et document de travail en neuropsychologie et neurolinguistique, Fasc. 2 #2, Université de Liège, 1987.
3. Ducarne de Ribaucourt, B.: *Rééducation séméiologique de l'Aphasie,* Masson, Paris, 1986.
4. Herrmann, M. & C.W. Wallesch: Psychosocial changes and psychosocial adjustment with chronic and severe non-fluent aphasia. *Aphasiology,* **3:** 513–526, 1989.
5. Howard, G. & Coll.: Factors influencing return to work following cerebral infarction. *J Am Ass,* **253:** 226–232, 1985.
6. Oder, W. & Coll.: Is aphasia an additional prognostic factor in ischemic stroke with regard to the severity of hemiparesis in the subacute stage? *Acta Neurol Scand,* **78:** 85–89, 1988.
7. Pariser, P. & C. Bergego: Les facteurs de prognostic des aphasies. *Rev Prat,* **36:** 981–984, 1986.
8. Weisbroth, S., N. Esibil & R.R. Zuger: Factors in vocational success of hemiplegic patients. *Arch Phys Med Rehabil,* **52:** 441–446, 1971.

COMPLEMENTARY BIBLIOGRAPHY

L'aphasie ou le bouleversement d'une vie, Mémoire d'orthophonie, Université de Besançon, année académique 1984–85.

Lavorel, D. & F. Michel: Bilan comportemental des handicaps du langage, Laboratoire de neuropsychologie, Hôpital Wertheimer, Lyon, 1984.

Sarno, J., M. Sarno & E. Levita: The Functional Life Scale (FLS). *Arch Phys Med Rehabil,* **54:** 214–220, 1973.

Seron, X.: Aphasie et neuropsychologie, Mardaga, Brussels, 1979.

Taylor, M.: A measurement of functional communication in aphasia (PCF de Sarno) *Arch Phys Med Rehabil,* **46:** 101–107, 1965.

Van Dunnen, S.: *Elaboration d'un test et propositions de traitement de la communication du patient aphasique dans la vie sociale,* Mémoire de graduat en ergothérapie, Iscam, 1983–84.

CHAPTER 14

THE PERSON WITH APHASIA AND THE LAW

F. COT AND R. DEGIOVANI,
WITH THE PARTICIPATION OF
T. HIRSBRUNNER

INTRODUCTION

Aphasia disrupts.

Aphasia causes personal disruption because it impairs expression of thought, and it confines the person to a closed universe.

Aphasia disrupts marriage when years, even decades, of life as a couple are shattered due to the inability to share one's ideas and feelings.

Aphasia disrupts the family as persons with aphasia quickly become strangers in their own homes, alienated from everyday life.

Aphasia disrupts the social environment since, without dialogue, in a few short months the circle of friends and neighbors dwindles away.

Aphasia also disrupts the person's relation with society.

How does the loss of language affect the link between people and society? How can men and women, with their multiple roles — worker, citizen, contributor to social security, proprietor, spouse — exist in society without the intermediary of language?

All those who come into professional or social contact with persons with aphasia are well aware that the impairment of normal expression of thought constitutes, beyond the human rupture, a generalized and severe limitation.

The onset of aphasia, accentuated by the invariable suddenness of the stroke that induced it, has a global effect, and spares virtually no aspect of the person.

However, within the population, despite a slight shifting of opinion, the plainly visible physical consequences tend to be better known than the communication disabilities. Most often, persons who acquire aphasia complicated by hemiplegia (an all too common condition) are basically viewed (and pitied) in terms of their physical disability. Language and cognitive deficits are downplayed, especially in people who have left or who have never entered the workforce. Onlookers' first impression, ignorance of the complexity, variety, and fluctuation of the problems, an unconscious fear of anything related to brain disorders, and the association between language impairments and psychological or mental illness, all this, undoubtedly explains the characteristic reactions of the general public and even, at times, of families and friends of persons with aphasia.

A priori, one can imagine that the *official* image of the person with aphasia must differ from this negative stereotype. In this chapter, we will focus our attention on the legal system, setting aside individual impressions of persons with aphasia (which can be read in other chapters of this volume). We will examine the *official* place of the person with aphasia in society, particularly in terms of the pertinent laws and regulations.

This description is certainly inseparable from society's view of a specific problem: That of communication. How is the individual with aphasia recognized and treated: This individual who, with his disrupted speech, can no longer participate as a full-fledged member of the community?

From the opposite point of view, how can the person with aphasia *function* in society? How can he respond at work, cut off from his primordial mode of communication, in his local bank, at the ballot box, at the notary, behind the wheel of his car? How can he perform daily activities, all of which have legal implications? This evaluation and reflection are by no means useless stylistic exercises, mainly because the relationship between people, language, and society forms an essential bond in our civilization. In our society, which is leaning more and more towards the service sector, i.e. towards human relations, the notion of communication is omnipresent, even if it often loses some of its basic meaning — that of dialogue between individuals. Furthermore, persons with aphasia constitute a group which is hardly negligible. Although there is no precise epidemiological data on aphasia, even in the United States[1], various estimates can serve to assess the social impact of aphasia.

PREVALENCE OF APHASIA IN THE UNITED STATES AND IN QUEBEC

The United States

In 1975, there were an estimated one million adults with aphasia in the country (*Resource Materials for Communication Problems of Older Persons, 1979 ASHA*). Moreover, Albert and Helm-Estabrooks[1] claim that there are:

- 85,000 new cases of post-stroke aphasia in the United States each year;
- 1.4 million patients with language disabilities and communication difficulties induced by trauma, as of 1982.

Quebec (Canada)

Between 1974 and 1978, there was an average of 2,300 cases of stroke treated annually (*L'intégration de la personne handicapée*, 1981). According to American studies (which are more abundant), aphasia is present in 20 to 30% [2,12] of strokes, which would result in at least 460 to 690 new cases in Quebec (with a population of over 6 million).

The ever-growing numbers, a result of improvements in the vital treatment of persons with stroke and brain injuries, are proof of the need to consider seriously the problem of the relationship between the person with aphasia and the society.

We will first examine how aphasia was viewed from a medicolegal standpoint at the time of its *discovery,* at the turn of the last century. We will then analyze the current situation in France and Quebec, with a brief mention of Switzerland.

AN OVERVIEW OF THE MEDICOLEGAL TREATMENT OF APHASIA

The First Aphasiologists

Authors in the late 19th-early 20th century were more preoccupied with the medicolegal aspects of aphasia than are researchers today. To quote Legrand du Saulle (in Martin[14]):

> "In some cases, persons with aphasia, while retaining their intelligence, are unable to execute a holograph, public or secret will." (See "The Legal protection of the Person with Aphasia" below).

Lutaud, in his *Manuel de médecine légale*[13] wrote that persons with aphasia find themselves in a very difficult situation in terms of executing their wills. In some circumstances, they are unable to leave a holograph will or a mystic testament (dictated by the testator to a third person). If they are unable to write, they find themselves in the same position as the deaf-mute, and are therefore unable to bequeath. By law, a will must be handwritten or dictated by the testator. A person may not bequeath by gestures nor by answering questions; all jurists concur on this queston.

Even the great Déjerine discusses the subject in his *Sémiologie des affections du système nerveux*[7] (Semiology of disorders of the nervous system). He discusses the intellectual abilities of persons with aphasia, which, he claims, vary widely between subjects:

> "To summarize, each case must be analyzed individually, based on a fastidious observation of the patient. These comments also apply to other medicolegal topics such as crimes, interdiction[1] and validity of a will, which might affect persons with sensory or motor aphasia".

Diller[9] considers that the doctor's role here is to determine whether the person with aphasia:

- is mentally sound;
- can comprehend;
- can communicate with others.

It is interesting to follow the evolution of the medicolegal literature over time. For example, in *Taylor's Principles and Practice of Medical*

[1] A legal process whereby a person's civil rights are removed.

Jurisprudence[19], a Bible in the field, two pages are devoted to aphasia in the 1948 edition, while in the 1984 edition aphasia is not mentioned at all. What are the implications of this change?

Over a century ago, the *Société de médecine légale de Paris* held a conference on the "interdiction of persons with aphasia"[11]. Subsequent to a report by Lefort, a lawyer, a committee of four doctors reached a conclusion, in substantia, based on the Civil Code. They defined three possibilities in terms of the residual capacities of the person with aphasia: Total interdiction, the designation of a legal adviser, and free administration of property. In all cases, the courts decide the fate of each person with aphasia individually, according to the extent of the disability.[2]

In the past two decades, interest by researchers, doctors, and speech pathologists has done much to expand the body of knowledge on aphasia. There are virtually hundreds of works devoted to the description and understanding of language mechanisms, along with the evaluation and treatment of aphasic deficits. Therefore, we can anticipate a greater number of references to aphasia in current legal texts than in those of the previous century, when, according to the members of the *Société de médecine légale,* research on aphasia had just begun. In fact, such references are not at all prevalent; to quote Jacques Ponzio, the law is aphasic with regards to aphasia!

The Medicolegal Literature

The medicolegal literature is pertinent here since, "legal medicine studies the relationship between the law and the various aspects of medical practice, whether curative or preventive".[8] Furthermore, "the cooperation of a doctor is needed to evaluate (amongst other things) the physical and mental condition of an individual".[8]

It seems as if the medicolegal literature is torn between two perspectives on aphasia:

- the link between aphasia and intelligence,
- the link between aphasia and mental health.

We have seen that Déjerine explored, from a medicolegal viewpoint, the intellectual capacities of persons with aphasia. He considers that intelligence to be intact in cases of pure aphasia (pure motor aphasia, and pure verbal blindness and deafness). In aphasia involving disturbance of internal language (global aphasia, sensorimotor aphasia, and Broca's aphasia) he claims the intellectual abilities are affected,

---

[2] Note the similarity with the modern solutions contained in the "Legal protection of persons with aphasia" below.

but often are only barely altered. In contrast, his contemporary, Pierre Marie, considers that aphasia is synonomous with *intellectual deficiency* in all cases, and that anarthria alone leaves intelligence intact.

Other authors have described aphasia as a form of mental illness. Lutaud, for example, mentions aphasia in the section "madness" in his *Manuel de médecine légale et de jurisprudence médicale.*[13] In fact, the law is more concerned with mental health. Section 901 of the French Civil Code states that "to make a will, or a gift inter vivos, a person must be of sound mind." Likewise, article 831 of the Civil Code of Lower Canada stipulates: "Every person of full age, of sound intellect, . . . may dispose of [his property] freely by will, without distinction as to its origin or nature . . ."

Thomas Szasz, author of *La loi, la liberté et la psychiatrie*[18], goes so far as to say that "the distinction between insane and sane is only significant in a legal context." We will thus continue with an examination of the psychiatric literature.

Psychiatric Literature

In psychiatry, even legal psychiatry, there is very little on the subject of aphasia. Nonetheless, manuals reveal that psychiatrists play a key role in the medicolegal field. They may be consulted as experts to evaluate the legal capacity of a person in cases where a will is contested, even if the testator is deceased! Since aphasia is most common in the elderly, this is an area of particular concern for persons with aphasia. Thus it is surprising that, given the weight of these decisions, there are so few references to persons with aphasia in the literature.

Nevertheless, *Psychiatrie médico-légale* by Porot and Bardenat[16] contains several informative references to persons with aphasia. For example:

> "It is very difficult to assess their mental aptitudes, errors on the positive or negative sides are quite likely, since such persons are impaired in their expression or comprehension (speech, writing, and reading)."

Principal Trends

Two types of analysis can be discerned in the medicolegal literature:

- a diagnostic approach,
- a case-by-case approach.

The first approach deduces legal capacity from aphasiological descriptions. For example, Porot and Bardenat[16] consider that "in total motor aphasia[7], there can be no valid form of will, the same applies for persons with Wernicke's aphasia." The second approach makes no *a priori* judgments; instead, it is based on individual assessment. Déjerine (see above) adopted this perspective.

There is an apparent incongruence in these viewpoints. Does aphasia affect the intellect? Should aphasia be classified as a mental disorder? What about the person's capacity to exercise civil rights such as succession, marriage, or divorce? Who should evaluate the person's capacity? There is little in the literature which clarifies the place of the person with aphasia in the legal system. Perhaps an examination of official legislation can shed more light on this issue.

APHASIA AND THE LAW

Here is a list of texts which make specific references to aphasia:

In France, apart from official tables which rate various problems (discussed below), to our knowledge, there is no text that contains the term "aphasia." A ruling on driver's licences determined that certain forms of aphasia represent disorders that are incompatible with the issuance or the renewal of a licence. Yet the new list, included in the ruling made on October 4, 1988, makes no mention of aphasia.

In Switzerland, the term "aphasia" does not appear in any legislation. A temporary removal of one's driver's licence only takes place subsequent to *information* supplied by the attending physician.

In Quebec, the same practice of suspension of one's driver's licence exists only if the attending physician informs the Quebec Automobile Insurance Board. Only one text explicitly refers to aphasia but the mention is restrictive. The Highway Safety Code (*Gazette officiele du Québec*, 1981) stipulates that:

> "A person who has Wernicke's sensory aphasia(!), apraxia or severe agnosia MAY NOT OBTAIN A PERMIT OF ANY KIND.
>
> "A person who aquires a disorder, apart from sensory aphasia, apraxia, or severe agnosia, which affects the higher intellectual functions, MAY NOT OBTAIN A DRIVER'S PERMIT EXCEPT FOR A PRIVATE VEHICLE WEIGHING LESS THAN 5500 Kg."

Furthermore, a new regulation (*Gazette officielle du Québec*, 1987) mentions that "neurological disorders inducing major disturbances to cognitive functions . . . are incompatible with driving a motor vehicle." Note that it is up to the physician to determine the extent of the disturbances to the cognitive functions.

Apart from these texts, it seems that there are no legal provisions which deal specifically with persons with aphasia. Aphasia is only rarely mentioned as such in court or in the doctrine. It is therefore difficult to find jurisprudence in this domain. Given the quasi-total legal void, we will examine various situations which could concern persons with aphasia in order to discern their place in the law and in society.

PERSONS WITH APHASIA AND THE LAW

Despite the dearth of legal references, persons with aphasia must interact with the law, since, like each of us, they have rights and obligations. In some cases, the law may even remove some or all of these rights.

The Legal Definition of Capacity

Capacity is defined as "the faculty granted by law to certain persons to engage in acts which have legal consequences".[15] "The faculty to conduct oneself in every aspect of life in society, and the full enjoyment of rights as a citizen constitute civil capacity".[14] More precisely, we are referring to the right to enter into contracts, to acquire, administer, and dispose of property, to engage in business, to marry, to testify in court, etc. "The law is concerned with tutorship and emancipation, and can even completely suspend legal capacity . . ." (ibid.) Incapacity can be defined as the legally imposed impossibility to exercise freely one's civil rights.

Of all these civil acts, jurists are most concerned with wills and testaments; this is the body of literature which contains the most references to aphasia.

The Capacity to Bequeath

Aphasia is mentioned by Lutaud[13] among the "principal pathological conditions that can be detrimental to the freedom of the testator's mind, and subsequently lead to invalidation." Legrand du Saulle (1865) also emphasizes that bequests by persons with aphasia may give rise to serious problems. He mentions the example of a 50-year-old person with aphasia who, despite his efforts to "assemble his words . . . was unfortunate enough to die before he could draw up, as best he could, his last will and testament." He adds that it is important that patients settle their successions before a notary and in the presence of witnesses. These two early texts stress the communication impairment of persons with aphasia.

More precisely, and for lawyers especially, the following points are essential to the ability to bequeath:

- understanding the nature and the consequences of the act;
- knowing the nature and the extent of one's property;
- knowing the heirs[4, 18].

There are two possible scenarios:

- the will is already drawn up, and it is contested (generally by the legal heirs who feel wronged);
- the will has yet to be drawn up.

When the will is contested (due to a conflict of interest), psychiatrists are often called in to determine before the courts whether the testator met the three criteria mentioned above, at the time the will was drawn up[6].

One may ask why the psychiatrist is considered an expert in this case. It is because actually, brain disorders fall under the category of psychiatry, specifically "neuropathology".[18] This fact is significant since it *categorizes* aphasia. In reality, the reliance on psychiatric expertise in court implies that persons with aphasia are not of sound mind, while the opinion of a neurologist relates more to functional and cognitive difficulties, such as the linguistic capacities of the patient. In fact, in this particular aspect of legal medicine, it would be more logical to solicit the opinion of a neurologist, together with that of qualified professionals who have had extensive contact with persons with aphasia, such as speech pathologists and neuropsychologists.

The most enlightening document available on the subject of aphasia is an article by Critchley entitled *Testamentary Capacity in Aphasia*[5]; the author is evidently familiar with persons with aphasia. He considers that a neurologist should be consulted as an expert to consider two separate issues:

- the will,
- the testator.

The Will

Is the will plausible? Did the patient disinherit the spouse and children and leave his inheritance to strangers or to charity? Is the content compatible with the intellectual aptitudes of the person in question? Critchley affirms that a long and complex will would seem unlikely given the difficulties of abstraction linked to most forms of aphasia except the least severe.

The Testator

If the testator is deceased, the neurologist must, according to his notes and specific knowledge of the patient, clarify the person's mental condition, his capacity in all spheres, and his ability to comprehend language. Furthermore, he will take into account fluctuations in the intensity of the symptoms and possible accompanying behavioral disorders. Neurological results are also significant, including the presence or absence of diffuse, extensive or multiple cerebral lesions, and the combination of senility and aphasia.

If the testator is alive, the neurologist can examine the person at will, and, as Critchley states[5], can seek the opinion of other consultants. We consider that this would be an appropriate point for speech pathologists to intervene. A language examination can supplement neurological observations by pinpointing the possibilities and limits of the person with aphasia in terms of oral and written comprehension. Such an assessment can also clarify preferential forms of communication. The severity of each case, rather than the aphasiological diagnosis itself, seems to be primordial. Finally, other factors such as the tendency towards fatigue, perseverations, and the variability of the symptoms can be taken into account. We strongly believe that the examination should cover not only the linguistic capacities of the patient but should also assess the overall patterns of communication. A pragmatic assessment would be highly pertinent here.

The Civil Code of Lower Canada (an old term for the area of Canada presently known as Quebec), which applies in Quebec, specifies three possible forms of wills available to persons with aphasia. (Art. 842):

- the holograph will, wholly written by the testator, which requires neither the presence of notaries nor witnesses;
- the authentic will, written by a notary, and dictated and signed by the testator in the presence of two witnesses or another notary;
- the will in the form derived from the laws of England (which greatly resembles the mystic will of the French Civil Code). This will is in writing and signed by the testator or another person for him in his presence and under his express direction, in the presence of at least two competent witnesses.

Porot and Bardenat[16] consider the

> "authentic will, executed in the presence of a physician capable of evaluating the degree of lucidity of the subject, the only acceptable will for persons with aphasia."

Note that wills in authentic form cannot be dictated by signs (Art. 847), but only by word of mouth, or by written instructions by the testator. Although the law provides for people with hearing impairments but not for persons with aphasia, Article 852 of the Civil Code can apply to persons with aphasia:

> "Deaf mutes capable of understanding the meaning of a will and the manner of making one, and all other persons, whether literate or not, whose infirmity has not rendered them incapable of so understanding or of expressing their intentions, may dispose of property by will in the form derived from the laws of England, provided their intention and the acknowledgment of their signature or mark are manifested in presence of witnesses."

Critchley[5], followed by Benson[2], described a procedure which seems to protect adequately persons with aphasia. He suggests the presence of a neurologist, a consultant (unspecified), and a justice of the peace. Several precautions are taken so as to consider the variability of the symptoms, the presence of perseverations, paraphasias, written comprehension deficits, etc.

These steps include:

- postponing the drawing up of the will until the testator's mental state improves;
- wording the will in as brief and simple manner as possible;
- repetition of the questions in order to ensure that the testator has clearly expressed his wishes;
- slow rereading of the will to the patient;
- unanimous agreement on the fact that the person with aphasia understands and approves of the contents of the will.

Clearly, these measures demand much time and patience. They do, however, take into account the particularities of aphasia. Furthermore, they allow for the comprehension and expression deficits common in persons with aphasia, while simultaneously relating fully to the person's actual capacity to make sound judgments. Testaments and wills have long interested us, partly due to their near-universal validity, and partly because of the extensive literature on this topic. Wills, however, are merely one aspect, albeit a meaningful one, of the total capacity to administer one's property.

Legal Protection of Persons with Aphasia

For the past few years, social workers and other professionals have become aware of a growing phenomenon which is sad, but true: Abuse of the elderly. This abuse includes financial exploitation as well as physical or psychological violence, severe mistreatment, and even rape. In the United States, the number of abused elderly persons varies, according to one study, from half a million to 2.5 million. Women over 75 are particularly affected by this problem. Furthermore, the major source of violence against the elderly is within the family. A report entitled *Protection of the Elderly*, published in Manitoba in 1982, is quite informative[17].

We are not citing these facts in the interest of sensationalism, rather they provide a backdrop for the discussion that follows. It seems to us that these data are particularly pertinent for persons with aphasia. The Canadian Charter of Rights and Freedoms states that: "Any elderly or disabled person has the right to protection against all forms of exploitation" (Art. 48). In the United States, as well as in Canada, the law attempts in various ways to ensure protection for those who are unable to stand up for their rights or administer their property. Since a person with aphasia is, on the one hand, vulnerable to exploitation of his person and property, and on the other hand, has difficulty with everyday administrative tasks, (e.g. paying bills), it is useful to examine the means of legal protection available to adults in France and Quebec.

Here again, we found that the law does not specifically provide for persons with aphasia. Aphasia as such does not appear in official legislation and it is only through extrapolation that one can find legal situations that are applicable to the experiences of persons with aphasia.

In France, there are three available forms of legal protection:

- **Legal protection** per se: a temporary and immediate measure, initiated by the attending physician upon a psychiatrist's recommendation. The person protected retains his capacity, but acts contrary to his interest can be annulled.
- **Curatorship:** an intermediary step, whereby the person protected retains the right to administer his property, but may not dispose of it.
- **Guardianship** implies total incapacity of the person, who is deemed an interdict[3] . The person must be represented by his tutor in all civil acts. Guardianship implies the recognition of a chronic irreversible disability which severely hampers the expression of free will.

Article 490 of the law dealing with the rights of interdicts, enacted on January 3, 1968, states that when mental faculties are altered by an illness, deficiency, or debility due to age, it is in the best interests of the person to resort to legal protection. These measures are applicable to physical disabilities, "if these disabilities impair the ability to express free will". The guardianship judge decides which measure to apply, on the basis of recommendations by experts in the medical field.

In Switzerland, legislative provisions are identical to the measures above. Aphasia is not mentioned in the legislation. However, many laws are currently under revision, and certain consultants are proposing that legislation be introduced that would distinguish between psychiatric or aphasia and other disorders.

Similarly, in Quebec, the "Public Curator Act" provides for three forms of legal protection which are applied when a person is judged to be incompetent as a result of illness, deficiency, or debility due to age[4]. These forms consist of curatorship, tutorship, or protection by an advisor to the person of full age.

- **Advisor to the person of full age:** provided for a person who, although generally and habitually able to care for himself, requires,

[3] A person of legal age who is deemed incompetent by the courts.

[4] This illness, deficiency, or debility must affect the mental faculties, or the person's physical ability to express his free will.

for certain acts or for a certain time, to be assisted or advised in the administration of his property.

- **Tutorship:** the person is unable, either temporarily or partially, of caring for himself and administering his property.
- **Curatorship:** this is the strongest form of protection. It involves only cases where the inability[5] to care for oneself and administer one's property is total and permanent.

On the basis of medical and psychosocial reports, the courts evaluate the ability or inability of the person, and then determine the protective supervision. The application for the institution of protective supervision is made either by the person himself, by a relative or by a person showing special interest in the person, or by the Public Curator. It is important to note that the law calls for periodic review of the person's file, in order to ascertain that the protection remains adequate.

The courts can institute protective supervision for a person or property, as well as a person and his property. They can also determine which acts the person is capable of performing on his own or with the help of his tutor, and for which acts he must be represented.

Furthermore, Quebec offers a new and original procedure: The **mandate**, which allows any able adult to avoid falling under legal protection if they do become incompetent. In the eventuality of one's inability it is, in fact, possible to designate beforehand a trusted person (or persons) who will then be responsible, if necessary, for major decisions regarding property and the person. The mandate can be notarized, or even drawn up in the presence of witnesses. This deed is particularly pertinent to persons with aphasia, and can serve anyone with foresight. Note that a simple proxy form becomes void as soon as a person is judged to be incompetent, while the mandate comes into effect under identical circumstances (*Public Curator Act L145*).

- One can observe that, in order to protect the person, the law deprives him of the capacity to exercise certain rights (e.g. the right to adminster property, or the right to consent to medical treatment), or even all of his rights. This is the cost the person must pay in order to have a legal representative.
- Of all the criteria relevant to the institution of legal supervision, legislators have only considered conditions which *impair mental faculties or the physical ability to express one's will.* When aphasia

[5] Inability (or incompetence) implies that a person can no longer attend to himself and/or his property. Legal recognition of this state, whereby the court institutes legal protection is known as interdiction.

exceeds simple problems of expression, must it then be categorized as a mental disorder?

- It is worth questioning the manner in which medical and psychosocial evaluations are performed. In order for a decision of such magnitude to be as effective and as precise as possible it: ". . . must be founded on a serious functional analysis of the person, one which encompasses all aspects of his social and interpersonal activities."[10]

ARE PERSONS WITH APHASIA DISABLED?

In the Western world, over the last few decades, a generally vast and complex system of benefits, pensions, and allowances has arisen in order to meet the needs of the elderly and the disadvantaged. Virtually every possible situation is covered by the web of social assistance. Nonetheless, we shall examine whether the medico-administrative regulations have provided for persons with aphasia. We shall also determine the place of such persons in the social aid network.

Statistically, aphasia tends to appear more frequently in people over age 60. Subsequently, many people are already retired when they acquire aphasia. These people are receiving old age pension, and their condition does not incur a loss of income.

Yet younger people, also, acquire aphasia. Some even quite young indeed (those who were injured during traffic or work-related accidents), and in the midst of their professional lives. For a time (officially up to three years in France, and two years in Switzerland), the standard provisions dealing with work stoppage apply, without mention of the person's specific disability. Daily indemnities are paid out without the person having to describe the precise nature and extent of the language deficit. The apparent impossibility of a return to work is often attributed to trauma, or to the initial illness, related motor difficulties, other neurological problems (e.g. epilepsy), or the need for extensive medical treatment. In a sense, the aphasia seems to get left by the wayside from the start.

The situation changes concurrently with the stabilization of the pathological state. In the case of stroke, the initial condition may improve with proper patient management. It is believed that the illness later gives way to a static residual condition, although gains or adaptations are still possible with rehabilitation. This condition is then considered to be a chronic and often irreversible deficiency. In fact, it is the status of the person with aphasia that changes, from that of a person with a temporary illness to that of a person with a permanent disability.

In France, in administrative terms, this change coincides with intervention by the *Commission technique d'orientation et de reclassement professionel*[6], or COTOREP. This committee, created by the "Orientation Act," on June 30, 1975, has a dual role:

- to evaluate the ability to work, as well as to *declare* the person disabled;
- to set the disability rate.

Article L.323–10 of the Labor Code states that a disabled worker is anyone whose possibilities of obtaining and preserving employment are significantly reduced following a deficiency or diminishment of the person's mental or physical capacities. This surely applies to many persons with aphasia. Their possibilities of retaining a job are limited, even nonexistent (despite certain optimistic statistics). To the contrary, one reason for this difficulty is that, in addition to the language impairment, persons with aphasia also have problems coping with complex interactional situations (Box 1).

Box 1

Mr. P. recovered adequate oral and written language, in terms of the classic language assessment scales. However, he was unable to grasp rapid and complex conversation between three people. Moreover, he could not listen and take notes simultaneously. Despite his success in laboratory tests, he was unable to return to his clerical job.

How does this law apply to persons with aphasia? To use the terms of the Labor Code, is aphasia a diminishment of physical or mental capacities?

- For those persons, few and far between, who show no signs of other disabilities, only the heading "mental disability" can grant them recognition by COTOREP as a person with a disability.
- *Fortunately*, in a sense, aphasia is often accompanied by other more visible disabilities, primarily hemiplegia, but also visual impairments, (in particular hemianopsia) and even epileptic seizures. In those cases, aphasia falls under the category of a "physical disability."

In a society which is quite willing to overemphasize physical disabilities, these problems, which are sometimes only secondary to severe aphasia(the key reason why professional activity cannot be resumed) are better acknowledged and entitle the person to disability *benefits*.

[6] Technical Committee for Professional Orientation and Reclassification.

The second role of COTOREP allows for a refinement of the official view on aphasia, since it involves determining the level of disability. We shall consult the ratings tables which are employed, in particular the scale of military disability pensions. Although this table was first proposed in 1918, it is still used as a reference by COTOREP. Here is how it regards aphasia:

APHASIA (global aphasia is exceptionally rare)

a)	with speech difficulties without considerable alteration of internal language abilities	10 – 30%
b)	sensory aphasia with alteration of internal language abilities	60 – 100%
c)	with the inability to communicate with others (alteration of internal language)	60 – 80%

Possible addition of mental deficits.
The rate of 60–80 mentioned above is valid when the aphasia is isolated.
If hemiplegia is also present, a rate of 20 will be added.

HEMIPLEGIA

d)	with aphasia	100%

From this official table, we can deduce the following:

- The notion of “internal language” seems to be the key element which differentiates mild and severe aphasia. Yet this notion is particularly vague and, at the very least, difficult to substantiate. It hardly seems to be an effective means of ensuring objectivity in the definition of the degree of incapacity.
- Moreover, does the difference between the rates for sensory and expressive aphasia mirror clinical reality? Moreover, how are impairments to written language — a virtually isolated deficit that may preclude a return to work — considered?
- The notion of “impossibility of communicating with others” has clear definitional problems.

An analysis of the table above clearly reveals that the assessment of the degree of disability urgently needs to be updated and better defined.

There are two other scales in use in France:

- the table of incapacities in common law (the Insurance Scale-19/06/82 Medical Examination); this table seems to be more attuned to reality, perhaps due to its approach and despite (or due to) its simplicity:

e)	aphasia: an impairment of varying degree to verbal expression, but not affecting comprehension of oral and written language	10–35%

f) with comprehension deficits which may preclude communication 40–95%

- the Social Security scale, which, in contrast, virtually ignores aphasia:

"Associated troubles[7] (for example aphasia, or sharp and chronic pain) which may coexist with motor impairments, must be evaluated separately."

What a smooth denial of a problem which actually affects the most profound aspects of an individual's personality!

Generally, one can note the relative insignificance of the rates allocated to aphasia, especially if one takes into account that 80% represents a key cutoff point for persons with disabilities. The rate of 80% allows persons to receive their disability cards, which are issued by COTOREP. This card grants the holder several *advantages*, particularly financial ones. Yet persons with *simple* aphasia never receive a rate which reflects their disability, although those persons may be severely cut off from life.

In the near future, the very minimum we can hope for is that the severity of the problems of persons with aphasia will finally be adequately assessed, and that the status of a person with a disability will be granted even in cases where aphasia occurs in isolation.

In Quebec, in a chapter that deals specifically with "Communication Problems," the C.S.S.T.[8] provides the following table in the annotated regulations on the table of corporeal injuries:

Class 1 Language impairment which slightly interferes with daily activities	15%
Class 2 Comprehension, but insufficient communication to engage in ordinary activities	40%
Class 3 No comprehension and unintelligible or inappropriate expression	70%
Class 4 No comprehension and an inability to communicate through language	100%

In Switzerland, jurisdiction lies either with Disability Insurance (AI), in case of illness, or with the *Swiss National Insurance Union* (CNA) in case of accident. The criteria for establishing disability and for fixing the disability rate are roughly similar to those found in

[7] with hemiplegia

[8] Commission de la santé et securité au travail (Health and Security at the Board of Workplace) a provincial organization that is responsible for evaluating injuries resulting from accidents at work, or occupational illness.)

France. There are differences between cases of illness and accident. Decisions by the CNA tend to be more favorable. Yet once the pension is established, benefits for care and the reimbursement of medical expenses are only granted if the earning capacity of the person has visibly improved, or if the person retained his former earning capacity.

OFFICIAL RECOGNITION OF APHASIA AS A DISABILITY

The *Canadian Charter of Rights and Freedoms*, proposed in April 1982, prohibits any discrimination against persons with disabilities, regarding access to goods and services — particularly transport. In Quebec, the law providing for the rights of persons with disabilities defines these persons as follows:

> "Any person limited in the performance of normal activities and who, in a significant and persistent fashion, has a physical or mental deficiency, or who regularly uses an orthesis, a prosthesis or any other means of compensation for a disability".

We understand that the person with aphasia is also included in this definition. We appreciate the degree to which this type of disability is poorly understood (Box 2). In fact, there is presently no formal procedure which grants persons with aphasia recognition as persons with disabilities. Of course, steps such as an application for an income tax credit due to disability allows the person to be officially recognized as a disabled person by the Minister of Revenue. Moreover, visits to a clinic such as the CLSC[9], renewals of a driver's licence after suspension due to illness, and membership in an association for persons with aphasia can also represent indirect recognition of the status of a disabled person.

Box 2

Ms. C., 35, has aphasia. Her face is slightly distorted by a paralysis which also distorts her speech. (Her speech, however, remains comprehensible, and no other sign of aphasia is manifested). She occasionally loses her balance. She goes for walks and once an overeager guard witnessed the woman's loss of balance and crudely insinuated that she was inebriated (it was 4 P.M.). Stunned, the woman tried to explain, but received this reply: "You also talk like a drunk!" Naturally, Ms.C.'s shock intensified her speech impairment. In response to her attempts to clarify matters, followed by an outburst, the guard, casually observed by passersby, restrained Ms. C. until the police arrived. The police acknowledged their blunder and apologized. However, they added "but next time, be careful how you act. People might get the wrong impression!"

[9] Local Community Services Centre (in Quebec)

Nonetheless, the issue of disability and aphasia is not clearcut. Indeed, is it desirable to achieve recognition of aphasia as a disability? The book *A Study of Prejudice in the Evaluation of Disabilities* by Bégué-Simon[3] contains interesting ideas on the topic. For example:

"As long as categories are not defined, we cannot begin to count and subsequently to appreciate the severity of the difficulties of certain individuals, or determine the quality of resources needed to sufficiently diminish the problems."

The classification of impairments, disabilities, and handicaps, published in 1980 by the World Health Organization (WHO), is based on the following formula:

ILLNESS→IMPAIRMENT→DISABILITY→DISADVANTAGE (HANDICAP)

WHO defines these notions as follows:

- impairment corresponds to any loss of substance or alteration of a psychological or anatomical structure or function (at the organic level);
- disability consists in any partial or total reduction (resulting from an impairment) of the capacity to perform an activity in a certain fashion or to the extent that is considered normal or human (the personal level);
- the social disadvantage or handicap resulting from an impairment or a disability which limits or precludes the performance of normal activities, *taking into account age, sex, and social and cultural factors.*

From this perspective, the disability is linked to the situation: A person can be 100% disabled for a certain activity, and 0% for another. For example, a person with aphasia may be totally unable to request information over the phone, but may succeed at the same task when at the counter of the bus terminal. In the former case, the functional deficit cannot be compensated for, and the disability is evident. In the latter, the disability can be overcome, and the task is feasible.

We therefore consider that simple labelling will be of little advantage to the *silent minority*, i.e. persons with aphasia. We feel that, beyond categorization, or an index of global severity, persons with aphasia require an evaluation of functional deficiencies along with functional capacities. Certain organizations (such as the *Montreal Urban Community Transport Commission*) are wisely examining cases on an individual basis. There is a fine illustration of this method in the *Eligibility Policy for Adapted Transport for Persons With Disabilities*, published by the Quebec Ministry of Transport:

> "Appreciable differences are revealed in the evaluation of the difficulties of transport for persons with identical disabilities . . . A pre-established chart listing the various factors to be considered . . . cannot allow one to reach automatic decisions, uniform across Quebec, similar to a mathematical formula."

Therefore, we do not propose further constraining legislation; instead, we recommend the implementation of several measures to promote the social integration of persons with aphasia.

- Currently, only physical or mental impairments are taken into account in the legal and medicolegal texts. It is high time for the recognition of *cognitive* difficulties, well illuminated by recent scientific works. These disturbances include language troubles as well as mnesic and more general instrumental deficits linked to brain injury.
- Recognition by the medical world, in particular by expert doctors, of aphasia as an essential problem. This would call for a radical modification of the notion of deficit, which is currently too directly tied to the physical nature of disability.
- In the same vein, a disability scale taking into account cognitive difficulties (including language) should be introduced as soon as possible. This table should correspond with the latest medical and scientific findings in the field.
- A case by case approach would allow for precise decisions in this complex area. Even if problems are sometimes similar, each person experiences aphasia differently due to his individual communication background. The diagnosis can therefore neither be generalized nor simplified. It is inconceivable to deprive a person with aphasia of certain or all of his civil rights on the mere basis of an aphasiological diagnosis. Likewise, it would be unfair to prematurely ask a person with aphasia for his *free and enlightened* consent on the basis of his apparent *normality* alone.

At any rate, over and above these measures, the major goal is to sensitize society in general. We have obviously not touched upon all of the legal aspects which affect persons with aphasia in their daily lives. Issues we were forced to omit due to the lack of space, include the right to information, informed consent to medical treatment, and the protection of personal rights in health-care establishments. Yet of all the situations described above, it becomes evident that persons with aphasia do not have a clearcut place in the legal system. Aphasia is practically absent in official texts, and a person with aphasia can only be considered to exist legally in terms of assimilation with other groups in the population such as people who are incapacitated or have mental illnesses, or even the insane. In all cases, the image of the person with aphasia is severely distorted, the initial deficit becomes complicated by society's vague and deprecating attitude. In fact, one of the objectives of this volume is to contribute to a better knowledge of persons with aphasia and to a better understanding of their problems.

REFERENCES

1. Albert, M.L. & N. Helm-Estabrooks, Diagnosis and Treatment of Aphasia, part 1. *JAMA*, **259:** 1043–1210, 1988.
2. Benson, F.D., Psychiatric Aspects of Aphasia, *Br J Psychiatry,* **123:** 555–566, 1973.
3. Bégué-Simon, A.M., *De l'évaluation du préjudice à l'évaluation du handicap,* Masson, Paris, 1986.
4. Camps, F.E., *Gradwohl's Legal Medicine,* John Wright and Sons, Bristol, 3rd ed., 1976.
5. Critchley, M., Testamentary Capacity in Aphasia, *Neurology,* **11:** 749–754, 1961.
6. Davidson, *Manuel de psychiatrie médico-légale,* Ronald Press, New York, 1952.
7. Déjerine, J., *Sémiologie des affections du système nerveux*, Masson, Paris, 1914.
8. Desmarez, J.J., *Manuel de médecine légale à l'usage des juristes,* P.U.F., Paris, 1967.
9. Diller, Th., Some Medico-Legal Aspects of Aphasia, *J Nerv Ment Dis*, **21:** 292–297, 1894.
10. Groupe d'études sur les questions juridiques: L'aspect juridique des soins dispensés aux personnes souffrant d'incapacité mentale: la capacité, la prise en charge des intérêts et la protection des droits. *Santé Mentale au Canada,* 7–13, 1987.
11. Lefort, M.J., *Remarques sur l'interdiction des aphasiques,* Vol. 38, Société de Médecine Légale, Paris, 2nd series, 1872.
12. Leske, M.C., Prevalence Estimates of Communication Disorders in the U.S. Language Hearing and Vestibular Disorders, *A.S.H.A.,* **23:** 229-237, 1981.
13. Lutaud, A., *Manuel de médecine légale et de jurisprudence médicale*, Lauwereyns, Paris, 3rd ed. 1881.
14. Martin, E., *Précis de médecine légale*, Doin, Paris, 2nd ed., 1938.
15. Pagé, D., *Petit Dictionnaire du Droit Québécois et Canadien,* Fides, Montreal, 1975.
16. Porot, A. & Ch. Bardenat, *Psychiatrie médico-légale,* Maloine, Paris, 1959.
17. Shell, D.J., Protection des personnes âgées, **in** *Étude sur les personnes âgées maltraitées,* Senior Citizens' Council of Manitoba, 1982.
18. Szasz, T., *La loi, la liberté et la psychiatrie,* Payot, Paris, 1963.
19. *Taylor's Principles and Practice of Medical Jurisprudence*, J. & A. Churchill, Bournemouth, 1948.

COMPLEMENTARY BIBLIOGRAPHY

Ruling of July 21, 1954 (France)
Ruling of October 4, 1988 (France)
Canadian Charter of Rights and Freedoms, 1982.
International Classification of Impairments, Disabilities, and Handicaps, 1984, I.S.E.R.M.-W.H.O., Paris.
Civil Code of Lower Canada

French Civil Code
Gazette officielle du Québec, December 30, 1981, p. 5631.
Gazette officielle du Québec, June 10, 1987, p. 3352.
Le Curateur Public, I.S.B.N. 2-550-17526-3, Bibliothèque nationale du Québec, 2nd quarter, 1987.
Public Curator Act and amending the Civil Code and other legislative provisions (Bill 145).
L'intégration de la personne handicapée, État de la situation, 1981, Les conférences socio-économiques du Québec.
Politique d'admissibilité au transport adapté, 1983, Ministère des Transports. Quebec government.
Réglement annoté sur le barème des dommages corporels, Commission de la santé et de la sécurité au travail, I.S.B.N. 2-551-06838-X, Bibliothèque nationale du Québec, 2nd quarter, 1987.
Resource Materials in Communications Problems and Behaviors of The Older American, 1979, A.S.H.A.

CHAPTER 15

ETHICAL-MORAL DILEMMAS IN APHASIA REHABILITATION

M. TAYLOR SARNO

INTRODUCTION

Before World War II, aphasia rehabilitation for civilians was virtually unknown. Since that time, speech-language pathologists have worked with many aphasic persons in private practice, hospital, and rehabilitation medicine settings. The actual number of persons with aphasia who have received assessment and/or treatment is unknown, but it is believed that the treated represent only a small percentage of those who became aphasic through the years. It is estimated that there is a pool of about one million Americans who have acquired aphasia[9]. The observations to follow are based upon experience with aphasia rehabilitation in the United States.

There are ethical-moral issues of considerable magnitude posed by the clinical management of persons with aphasia. Most of these issues have barely been identified or explored. The most salient ethical questions concern matters such as the selection of patients for treatment (i.e., how do we determine which patients will "benefit" from treatment?), patient autonomy (i.e., is the patient included in the determination of his/her rehabilitation regimen?), the setting of rehabilitation goals (i.e., how are the goals of aphasia rehabilitation, including treatment termination, determined?), and the allocation of rehabilitation resources (i.e., are current reimbursement policies/practices adequate to meet needs?). The comments contained in this essay are intended to call attention to the necessity for giving these issues high priority status in all aspects of aphasia rehabilitation management. To explore this topic, however briefly, it is necessary to review certain observations about the impact of aphasia on the person.

APHASIA AND THE PERSON

Many of the chapters in this book have supported the idea that it is insufficient to describe aphasia as exclusively a "neurological problem," "linguistic deficit," or "speech-language pathology." The condition of aphasia should not be limited by a definition that separates the language pathology from the person. As has been pointed out, there is a strong bias in the literature to view language pathology as consisting only of impairment rather than adaptation symptoms[7]. Although the underlying cause of aphasia is the pathology of neural structures essential for normal communication processing, it could be argued that it is a "disorder of person" rather than a "disorder of language."

Aphasia is not an organ, a tumor, a foreign body, or other entity that can be removed from the person for examination. The onset of aphasia produces a sudden, profound alteration of the person that immediately sets off a chain of attitudinal reactions to illness, disability, sense of self, ability to cope with being socially different, feelings of loss, the lowering of self-esteem, and possible depression in the face of impaired human behavior, most of which are based on premorbid personality structure and experience. All of this is compounded by the real social and vocational limits imposed by the communication impairment as well as the severe social isolation that most people with any degree of aphasia generally experience.

For the most part, aphasia rehabilitation research has not been responsive to the "person" dimension of aphasia nor to the relationship of linguistic impairment to non-linguistic variables, often making research results irrelevant to the issues which surround aphasia treatment and recovery. The aphasia clinician has access to a large body of information pertaining to the classification, localization, neurolinguistic research, and treatment techniques but little information relevant to the consequences of the communication disorder on the person. This virtually exclusive focus on the communication disorder itself has tended to obscure the ethical-moral questions that are inevitably presented by a condition like aphasia.

Perhaps the most important reason why these issues have been neglected in aphasia rehabilitation relates to the fact that historically the field of biomedical ethics has been concerned primarily with the seemingly more urgent issues of high tech acute care medicine. Since aphasia is generally a chronic condition, it "lacks the visibility and fascination of the high tech dramas played out in acute care settings"[(6)].

One of the most important differences between the organization and practice of acute and rehabilitation medicine has to do with the conceptualization of the role played by those who provide and those who are the recipients of health care. These differences are embodied in the traditional medical model and associated with acute health care, on the one hand, and the team model that is fundamental to the practice of rehabilitation medicine on the other. It goes without saying that the marked contrast between these two philosophies of care is readily apparent, for example, in the goal setting process inherent in each mode of practice.

As is well known, the dominant clinical model today is biomedical and leaves little room for the social, psychological, and behavioral dimensions of illness. This traditional medical model is generally limited to identifying the characteristics of diseases, their etiology, pathology, and manifestations. But long-term chronic disability like aphasia and its associated physical, psychological, and social consequences requires that practitioners take a view of patient care that transcends the medical model. What is needed is an understanding of the human and social consequences of a chronic disorder. The conventional model is characterized by the provision of acute/restorative care through clinical procedures such as surgery, drugs, and the laying on of hands. In the traditional medical model, the pathology is almost entirely in the physical patient, leaving aside psychological and social considerations. The condition is acute and usually considered transient. The assumption is that if the patient complies with physicians' orders, he will be cured. The goal of this model is to save lives or to cure. It does not consider many of the far-reaching psychological consequences of illness.

In the medical model, the physician alone is the technically competent expert. As the ultimate authority and decision-maker, he is accountable for the patient's care that is administered through a chain of authority. For his part, the patient is expected to assume a "sick role" and is required to cooperate with the physician as a passive recipient of intervention. In this model, the goals and outcomes are clear-cut and absolute, the outcome is black or white. The patient is either dead or alive, there is pathology or there is not, or the patient is either cured or not cured. The patient's values and those of his family and community are not generally considered in the application of this medical model to health care participation.

In contrast, medical rehabilitation, which encompasses aphasia rehabilitation, is a "relativist," consequence-oriented system dealing with more open-ended goals and outcomes. For example, enhancing function, the *sine qua non* goal of rehabilitation, is especially variable and depends on a wide range of conditions. Medical rehabilitation concerns itself with the quality of life. It deals with the pathology in the patient as it interacts with his environment and society, with chronic conditions that are generally medically stable, but often permanent. The patient is expected to be an active participant in his medical care, his rehabilitation. In this model the physician functions as a team manager and educator working with a team of rehabilitation specialists. Intervention in rehabilitation medicine is "care driven" rather than "cure driven."

There is, of course, some overlapping between these two sharply contrasting health care models. In fact, some of the boundary lines between the traditional biomedical model and medical rehabilitation have recently begun to merge. Technological advances have pushed the biomedical model into areas where quality of life issues have emerged (i.e., trauma centers), and rehabilitation medicine has even become involved in some high tech interventions.

It is an interesting fact that physicians trained in the specialty of rehabilitation have, only with great difficulty, transcended the traditional medical philosophy, inculcated in medical schools; that is, concern with pathology and acute care therapeutics. It could hardly be otherwise. It is still true that rehabilitation medicine specialists are looked upon somewhat askance by their clinical and research colleagues in the traditional medical specialties as being "a little more than kin and less than kind" (Shakespeare, *Hamlet*, Act I).

The philosophy underlying rehabilitation medicine and the realities which shape its practice have highlighted the narrow (restrictive) limits of the traditional biomedical model. It has not been possible to apply the traditional model to a medical specialty whose goals include such considerations as individual needs, social roles, and the distinction between impairment and disability. Such notions as functional assessment and personal expectations are not considered in the biomedical model. It does not account for how two individuals with seemingly equivalent degrees and type of pathology may be so far apart with respect to the outcome of rehabilitation that one of them may be able to return to work and the other cannot. The multiple factors which influence rehabilitation outcome must be considered.

Patients, families, and health professionals have a wide range of interpretations for the term "recovery." Most patients do not consider themselves recovered unless they have fully returned to previous levels of language competence[13]. "Recovery" is a psychological perception and should not be confused with an objective evaluation of communication skills. In the final analysis, the true test of outcome in aphasia rehabilitation can only be assessed by patients' perceptions of the quality of their lives[11]. Traditionally, the specialty of rehabilitation medicine has concerned itself with the issues which relate to the disabling/handicapping effects of various neurological impairments and has long acknowledged that the ability of patients to function in their daily lives, the so-called activities of daily living, does not necessarily correlate directly with the extent of motor, sensory, and language impairment. An individual may manifest significant impairment without an equivalent degree of disability. This phenomenon is present in the individual with aphasia, where language tests may identify specific deficits which may or may not correlate with an individual's use of language for communication in everyday life, referred to as functional communication effectiveness[11].

PATIENT SELECTION

A distinguishing feature of rehabilitation practice in the United States is that practitioners choose their patients. Most of those who receive rehabilitation services are referred by their physicians. Once the referral is made, a decision is reached as to whether or not a patient is an appropriate candidate for rehabilitation services. Candidacy is based on the belief that the patient can "benefit" from the services.

For the patient with aphasia, the admission process may present a particularly difficult situation. There are no formal or public criteria governing the decisions to admit patients for rehabilitation services. The primary factors that influence access to treatment relate to potential for success, ability to pay, and the anticipated burden that might be placed on staff members in the patients' care. In this context, such factors as age can become singularly important. Younger patients may receive priority over older patients in access to rehabilitation on the basis that they will live longer than older candidates. This practice is particularly difficult for individuals with aphasia, who, more often than not, are members of the older age group and whose ability to "benefit" is generally not considered sufficient to warrant the cost of rehabilitation services. Using the "potential to benefit" as a selection criterion raises a number of ethical and moral questions. How is "benefit" defined? Is it in terms of improved speech or greater access to a written vocabulary? Adaptation and reintegration into the community in the absence of significant improvements in communication function? Could not the term "benefit" also be defined as the ability to assert one's self, one's autonomy, in new ways which contribute to the resurgence and reaffirmation of personhood? Are not rehabilitation goals more concerned with "quality of life" issues than the goal of "cure" inherent in acute medical care[10]? In many facilities in the United States, the primary criterion for admission is financial clearance. Also, since strong family support may enhance rehabilitation outcome, those in charge of the admissions process often give particular attention to the geographic and emotional availability of support persons. Patients who lack viable discharge plans may be refused. Since there are no courses, written materials, or other training devoted to explicating some of the moral dilemmas inherent in the patient selection process, biases may creep into the system in many ways. For example, many practitioners believe that maximum recovery from aphasia only takes place in the first three to six months post onset, an opinion which would disqualify the large number of aphasic patients who continue to make progress for periods of time well beyond that point. Third party payers generally do not reimburse aphasic patients for rehabilitation beyond the early stages of the post acute period. Furthermore, some third party payers require that patients seeking admission to rehabilitation programs must demonstrate vocational potential, believing that the restoration of the ability to work is the treatment goal. Needless to say, this criterion would render the majority of patients with aphasia ineligible for services.

Patients may never be told about the reasons for their rejection, leaving patient and family to speculate that the rejection for admission reflects a negative prognosis for recovery, or, the equally devastating idea that admission was denied because they are not worthy as a person of the opportunity to receive treatment. The morality of such practices is questionable, and greater efforts must be made to study the patient selection process for rehabilitation services and communicate the factors involved in the process to the public.

Several observers have noted that rehabilitation resources are scarce and usually made available only to selected individuals — the services tend to be more available to the more educated, affluent, assertive individual. Some have pointed out that those from less privileged circumstances may require additional rehabilitation resources in order to achieve a rehabilitation goal[3]. This is one of many inequities in medical rehabilitation which run parallel to inequities in the society at large. While we can do little about this we must be aware of these inequities and their effect on many disabled individuals.

SETTING GOALS

Both patient and care provider bring different individual values to the goal setting process, which can lead to conflict between provider and patient, patient and family, and family and payer. Unlike the practice of acute medicine, rehabilitation medicine encourages and supports a consideration of the values of all concerned, and this, almost by definition, means a lack of consensus.

The goals of aphasia rehabilitation are not standardized and must be based on considerations of the patient as an individual with his own unique demographic features, assets, and liabilities, living in a particular community and society, at a particular point in time. There are several sides to the problem. Should the goals relate to linguistic improvement alone? To adjustment to being a person with aphasia? To the person's return to work or the social setting? Should they relate to a presumed potential level of improvement? And who should set the goals: the patient, the family, the speech-language pathologist, the physiatrist? Who should be the ultimate authority on what reasonable goals should be set? If the acute care physician were to determine rehabilitation goals, he might dismiss the person with aphasia as a hopelessly disabled member of society for whom intervention of any kind would prove futile[10].

A host of dilemmas is presented by these conflicting views when considering treatment goals. The open-ended quality of aphasia rehabilitation forces a great deal of negotiation among the principal characters in the rehabilitation scenario, the patient, family, physician, and members of the rehabilitation team. Goal setting is ideally negotiated among the various participants, but the process can be very much influenced by the degree of power each has at different stages of the rehabilitation process. One way to help correct some of the imbalance often present in the goal setting process is to include another participant, such as an ombudsman[3].

When and how to terminate aphasia therapy constitutes another moral quandary. Whose standards and values should guide the continuing care? Where should rehabilitation medicine end and educational and social agency care begin? Can the termination of speech therapy for the person with aphasia be considered the equivalent of abandonment in the rehabilitation context[10]?

Values play an important role in the goal setting process, not only those of the patient and his family, but of health care team members as well. Rehabilitation, and aphasia rehabilitation in particular, will be obliged to reassess its goals and examine what ethical value systems will dictate its goal setting practices with the advent of new medical financing guidelines and systems. One hopes that policy makers will want more than a promise of simply Activities of Daily Living (ADL) gains, physical restoration, and an increase in noun vocabulary, and a gain in writing, and that goal setting will not be politicized by reimbursement tyranny.

Thus far, medical rehabilitation in the United States has been exempt from the Medicare Diagnostic Related Groups (DRG) system, allowing its open-ended goals to remain unchallenged. But this is only temporary until a fixed payment formula is agreed upon. Once this happens medical rehabilitation goals will become more sharply focused and will probably be forced to revert to a more traditional medical model limiting patient goals.

RESOURCE ALLOCATION FOR APHASIA REHABILITATION

While precise data are not available, it is generally believed that the number of persons with aphasia who might benefit from access to speech-language pathology services far exceeds the number who have received or are receiving treatment. Further, the prohibitive cost of private aphasia therapy and the severe restrictions limiting reimbursement for services make aphasia rehabilitation inaccessible for most people. It has become increasingly apparent that aphasia therapy must be intensive, comprehensive, and of long duration. The realization of this therapeutic ideal is hindered by the inadequate number of speech-language pathologists who possess the interest and expertise to work with aphasia and the grossly deficient availability of public funds to support such treatment. It is likely that this situation will not improve substantially until there is a considerable increase in the number of studies supporting the efficacy of aphasia rehabilitation and documenting the psychosocial impact of the disorder and the need for prolonged therapy.

PATIENT AUTONOMY

Aphasiologists know that while many persons with aphasia are competent to make decisions, they may be unable to express themselves sufficiently well to exercise their autonomy. Rehabilitation professionals are often faced with the challenge of trying to restore or encourage autonomous behavior in patients who are depressed or devastated by the severity of their impairments[1]. Surrogate decision makers such as a spouse or parent have similar problems adjusting to a patient's new identity and future limitations. The capacity for free, voluntary choices is often impossible in many severely impaired individuals with aphasia. Yet, aphasia therapists are challenged to explore different strategies in the hope of restoring the person's autonomy with whatever degree of persuasion or time is necessary. In the very early stages of aphasia, it is usually necessary to exercise some paternalism while the patient comes to terms with the nature of aphasic impairment.

THE SELF

It is essential that we understand the extent to which an acquired disability like aphasia affects a person's identity. The sense of self, combined with a sense of the purpose and meaning of life, contribute to this perception. Impairments, disabilities, and handicaps have different meanings to different individuals, and these values play an important role in all stages of recovery, rehabilitation, and reintegration into the community. "Understanding the self is not a matter of scientific or empirical knowledge that can be decided once and for all"[4]. In the Judeo-Christian philosophy there is an idea of "self" — a beginning, a middle, and an end. In rehabilitation, we work at helping the patient think about the "now." The self as now. What does the patient want for himself now? The activities that helped define the person are no longer there, or they are altered. The patient is a new self. A dynamically evolving self in a new relationship to its body and to other members of the community of similarly impaired individuals. The family also needs to evolve a new "self" [5].

Maslow[8] conceived of successful rehabilitation as a process of shifting from survival to self-actualization — a rationale for rehabilitation which is incompatible with the traditional mode. Yet, it has been noted that the disabled often have a reduced drive for self-actualization which, if rehabilitation goals do not take into account, may lead to failed rehabilitation efforts. Maslow pointed up the fundamental relationship between self-concept and the rehabilitation process, since self-actualization depends upon the individual becoming what he is capable of becoming. For many disabled patients, this means redefining the quality of life in an altered state. Many persons with aphasia have referred to an evolving identity from the preaphasia "self" to a new "self."

CONCLUSION

In a report about ethical challenges relating to chronic illness, Jennings et al.[6] aptly state, "existing policies of health care, financing, and priorities in medical education and research give short shrift to the quality of life goals of chronic illness. Chronic illness is a reminder of the universal frailty and uncertainty of the human condition." Chronic disability, like aphasia, is a moral challenge, because it forces us to confront the question of how a good society should accommodate the "expectable — but always unexpected — misfortunes that occur in everyone's life"[6]. The provision of care and social support for persons with chronic disabilities by those of us temporarily well and able-bodied acknowledges the bonds between the sick and the well, the young and the old, in a "community of common humanness and vulnerability"[6]. Given the history in this area, it will be very difficult to achieve this moral perspective. Those of us who have struggled with the ethical-moral issues associated with aphasia know well that it epitomizes the challenge posed by a chronic disorder.

REFERENCES

1. Caplan, A.L., Callahan, D. & Hass, J. (1987): Ethical and Policy Issues in Rehabilitation Medicine. *A Hastings Center Report.* (Supplement).
2. Cassell, E.J. (1991): Recognizing Suffering. Briarcliff Manor, NY: *A Hastings Center Report,* **21:** 24–31.
3. DeJong, G. (1986): Medical Models and Ethical Systems: The Role of Rehabilitation Goals. Discussion paper presented at the *Ethics & Rehabilitation Medicine Study Group* convened at the Hastings Center, Briarcliff Manor, NY, April 4, 1986.
4. Donnelly, S. (April 1988): Human Selves, Chronic Illness, and the Ethics of Medicine. Briarcliff Manor, NY: *A Hastings Center Report.*
5. Donnelly, S. (1989): Conference on Ethics and Rehabilitation. Chicago: *Rehabilitation Institute of Chicago.*
6. Jennings, B., Callahan, D. & Caplan, A.L. (February/March 1988): Ethical Challenges of Chronic Illness. Briarcliff Manor, NY: *A Hastings Center Report.*
7. Kolk, H. & Heeschen, C. (1990): Review: Adaptation Symptoms and Impairment Symptoms in Broca's. *Aphasiology,* **4:** 221–231.
8. Maslow, A.H. (1968): *Toward a psychology of being.* Princeton, New Jersey: VanNostrand Company.
9. National Institutes of Health. (1979): Aphasia: *Hope through research.* Bethesda, MD: NIH Publication # 80-391.
10. Sarno, M.T. (1986): *The Silent Minority: The Patient with Aphasia.* Hemphill Lecture. Chicago: Rehabilitation Institute of Chicago.
11. Sarno, M.T. (1991): Recovery and Rehabilitation, **in** M.T. Sarno (Ed.), *Acquired Aphasia* (2nd ed.) (pp. 521–0582). New York: Academic Press.
12. Sarno, M.T. (In press, 1992). Treatment in Aphasia: Research and Research Needs. Monograph (pp. xi-xvi). Bethesda, MD: National Institute on Deafness and Other Communication Disorders.
13. Yarnell, P., Monroe, P. & Sobel, L. (1976): Aphasia Outcome in Stroke: A Clinical Neuroradiological Correlation. *Stroke*, **7**, 514–422.

CHAPTER 16

ASSOCIATIONS FOR PERSONS WITH APHASIA

M.D. HUBERT AND R. DEGIOVANI

"Here, association, comforting" (R.D.)

"It's great, friends, here, I talk with people, I talk, I talk, I can finally talk, talk with MY words . . ."(J.G.)

"It's hard to get people to listen, they just don't listen. Here YES! YES!" (L.G.)

"I . . . am . . . talk . . . no. I was talking to myself with them . . .GOOD YES!" (M.C.)

"For me, the Association is an environment that stimulates integration into society . . . it also allows you to learn information about disabilities, it helps improve our lives." (F.P.)

"Helps to write, read, count . . . practice, practice." (G.R.)

"We need a group where we belong, a family, this the Association provides." (J.G.)

"So I can see that I'm not the worst off. It's good. I can help, me too, help someone." (R.L.)

"This can help us get organized. Confidence, to regain confidence, that's what we're experiencing right now. Like G. says, for him painting is a way to communicate . . . of expressing himself. They're all ways." (M.D.)

"The Association, not only socializing . . . no. no, news of the world, even knowledge even SCI-EN-TI-FIC!" (J.C.)

"The Association is also the person's loved ones . . . and all those who love us . . . The family especially, because they have many problems living with us. They are there with us, they help us, it's great. But they also talk to each other, they share all their problems . . . it's hard for them." (L.M.)

INTRODUCTION

Over the years, a plethora of associations have arisen to respond to the needs of persons and their families to meet and to exchange with others who are grappling with the same problem. Persons with aphasia and their families are no exception: Recently, and in significant numbers, they are seeking out social support.

Associations for people with physical or mental disabilities have been in existence for several decades. To name a few, there are associations for persons with paraplegia (France, 1933; Quebec, 1945), associations for persons with visual impairments (France, 1889; Canada, 1908), and for persons with mental disabilities (France and Canada, 1920).

It was only in the 1970s, even the 1980s, that associations for persons with *cognitive* deficits began to appear. These groups bring together persons with Parkinson's disease or Alzheimer's disease, children with dyslexia or dysphasia, and, of course, adults with aphasia. This rather late emergence is almost certainly due to society's dominant ideology which favors physical disabilities in particular, i.e. the visible, as opposed to the more discrete, fluctuating, complex, and therefore more arcane, cognitive disorders. The growing influence of international organizations such as the *World Health Organization* (WHO), is gradually shaping this ideology into a more global, universal approach towards medicine that takes into account human beings in their entirety. The proposal of the *International Classification of Diseases,* in 1978, was followed by the *International Classification of Impairments, Disabilities and Handicaps,* the *ICIDH,* in 1980. This represents a major turning point in the medical and paramedical world with regard to rehabilitation. It is just in the past few years that the notion of disability has tended to fade slowly in favor of the notions of deficits, incapacities, and handicaps which, since they emphasize the interaction between people and their environment, do much to allow for the identification of symptoms which are less overt[(1)]. Consider, for example, a cognitive disorder such as aphasia. It is well known that this cerebral syndrome was not discovered recently. The dawn of the 21st century marks 200 years of developments since the German physician Franz Joseph Gall (1758-1828), and others, studied this neurological phenomenon. In the introduction of a work devoted to aphasia[(2)], Professors François Lhermitte and André Roch Lecours trace the milestones in the history of our knowledge of aphasiology.

At any rate, while future practitioners have long been receiving the training necessary for a better comprehension, or at least a better recognition of the symptoms of aphasia, it was only late in the last century that the rehabilitation of the person with aphasia began to attract any particular attention. In *La rééducation de l'aphasie en France vers 1900*[(3)] Françoise Cot and Yves Joanette look back upon the work of Dr. André Thomas who, in 1895, recorded his first observations on rehabilitation. Half a century later, in 1948, Blanche Ducarne de Ribaucourt, a speech pathologist, first introduced rehabilitation in France at the *Clinique des maladies du système nerveux* (Clinic for disorders of the nervous system) under the tutelage of Professor Théophile Alajouanine[(4)] at the *Hôpital de la Salpêtrière*, in Paris.

Therapists' and physicians' interests gradually shifted from aphasia and the treatment of its symptoms to the life of a person with aphasia[(5)]. In a longitudinal study, Blanche Ducarne de Ribaucourt examined 600 case histories of persons with aphasia, the results of which were published in 1986[4]. Yet in an article that she published in 1967 along with Francois Lhermitte, she pays particular attention to persons with aphasia, and to the problems linked to their social and professional reintegration[6]. Doubtlessly influenced by her teachings, other practitioners have also become pragmatically (if we may use that term) involved with persons with aphasia, to assist them in founding these associations.

The first French association for persons with aphasia was founded in Lyon, in 1976. Since then, over 30 associations with the same interests have sprung up, and some have even formed federations. In May 1989, the "Premier congrès international des associations des personnes aphasiques et de leurs proches"[7] (The first international conference of associations for persons with aphasia and their families) was held in Brussels, organized by "Se comprendre" (Understanding One Another), the Belgian association for persons with aphasia. Several countries were represented: Belgium, France, the Netherlands, Germany, Spain, Switzerland, England, Canada, the United States, and Argentina. Although most of these associations have only been in existence for a few years, their history and individual experience attests to their significance. For persons with aphasia, their families, therapists, researchers, or authorities, the impact of these associations has become so great that this volume would not be complete without a description of these groups.

This chapter aims to provide a general overview of the main features that define associations for persons with aphasia and their families. First, we will present the reasons and conditions for their creation. Next, we shall describe the categories of members that belong to the associations. We will later summarize the objectives pursued by nearly all such organizations, as well as describe their activities. In addition, we will outline fundamental features of the management of these organizations. We will conclude with a discussion of certain sizeable challenges which pose a threat to the survival of these groups.

THE BIRTH OF AN ASSOCIATION: THE ROOTS OF ITS CREATION

Many associations, particularly the earliest ones, were founded as a result of the initiative of speech pathologists, social workers, psychologists, and occasionally physicians. These circumstances are surely not due to chance alone. In fact, they reflect a certain school of aphasia therapy: One which recognizes the complementary and indispensable role of the members of a multidisciplinary team.

For a long time, aphasia therapy had been strictly confined to attempts to restore to the persons with aphasia the language skills which they lost. Therefore, all efforts were aimed at improving the quantity and the quality of the speech and language to be reacquired. Naturally, this is the underlying goal of everyone who works with persons with aphasia.

Furthermore, therapy for family members of the persons with aphasia was formerly limited to a structured aid relationship, essentially coordinated by the therapist. Such an approach is indisputably necessary.

Yet a certain number of therapists were conscious of the futility of such exercises if a link had not previously been established between the knowledge acquired in therapy and the patient and the family's concrete everyday needs. For example, what good does it serve if persons excel in speech therapy if they are unable to speak outside of this limited context? This absurd situation is, unfortunately, not so infrequent! Moreover, how can the social and familial equilibrium be maintained if the person's setting is excluded from the overall treatment program? Families of persons with aphasia can understand speech therapy exercises and can observe the progress in a purely clinical context, yet they still perceive an immense communication gap between two vastly different worlds: the clinical world and everyday reality.

Scientifically speaking, this new approach has led to an increased awareness of nonverbal communication and to pragmatic orientations in speech therapy. In human and social terms, this methodology aims to allow persons with aphasia to reconnect with life, and to be reborn into their family environments despite the ever-present language disabilities. It is extremely important to create a climate that encourages a better comprehension of persons with aphasia by their families.

It is important that we keep in mind that even when patients with aphasia have made considerable progress in therapy, most often they have still lost confidence in their ability to express themselves. Their phonetic approximations, residual paraphasias, word-finding difficulties, problems understanding certain complex expressions or quickly analyzing information, (in short, all the traits that characterize the typical patient with mild aphasia), induce feelings of inferiority and insecurities towards potential conversation partners. As a result, persons with aphasia withdraw into themselves, and shun opportunities for dialogue, limiting their conversations to a few familiar expressions. What about the person whose aphasia is complicated by hemiplegia, diminished visual capacities, and significantly reduced communication, all of which cloud the prognosis of speech therapy? In such cases, the persons and their families experience feelings of extreme powerlessness as they confront the social isolation that rapidly encroaches. They subsequently succumb and silently accept their cross to bear.

Alas, these scenarios are all too frequent, and represent only a small portion of the global picture revealed in therapy. We must be sensitive to such problems. It is therefore urgent to find a way to create a final stage of speech therapy, one which promotes the use of speech and language in their primary function: communication.

Persons with aphasia and their families must undergo a lengthy process of social reintegration and full readaptation to their surroundings and to society. Several persons with aphasia refer to this process as "a second birth"[8] or "second life"[8]. From this perspective, it seems evident that the process is marked by a growing string of problems of everyday life that crop up one by one. Whether they involve people or situations, these challenges demand considerable flexibility on the part of the persons with aphasia and their families.

To plunge the persons with aphasia directly back into society, where they could frequently be exposed to ignorance, indifference, and rejection, would be highly destructive. The creation of associations for persons with aphasia has therefore been considered to be a springboard which allows persons with aphasia and their families to regain confidence, on the one hand, and to prepare for their return to daily routines. On the other hand, in total contrast yet still understandably, the association also provides a kind of sanctuary. Here people can enjoy needed leisure and support, away from the limitations and difficulties imposed by society. For some, this desire for protection has been a significant factor behind the creation of associations.

Other objectives have also occasionally surfaced during the founding of associations; these will be discussed later in the chapter. Generally, the two principal reasons mentioned above seem to be the determining factors in the creation of most associations.

In the space of a few years, such associations have multiplied. The magnitude of the phenomenon first struck us in May 1989, in Brussels, at the "First International Convention"[7]. Some associations boast dozens of members, and are founded upon elaborate and efficient structures that enable them to organize major gatherings. Others, less robust, limit themselves to meetings with relative regularity. In any case, regardless of their size, structure, or degree of sophistication, these associations all share the desire to remove the barriers of isolation that surround persons with aphasia and their families, while encouraging them to reestablish lost contact with the outside world.

THE COMPONENTS OF AN ASSOCIATION

The Members

Several categories of members take part in associations for persons with aphasia, and the relative importance of each of these groups affects the functioning of the organization.

Persons with Aphasia

Such persons usually constitute a majority among members, yet they do not form a homogeneous group. Here is an outline of three different categories of members with aphasia:

- Persons who view the association as a new work environment, since they had to leave their previous workplace at the time of their stroke. Despite their residual disabilities, they are often particularly active; they manage and coordinate the association as well as perform liaison with the public.
- Other persons whose symptoms have largely abated, and who only experience difficulties in specific situations such as group or telephone conversations. For them, social (but rarely professional) reintegration is complete. They are nonetheless drawn to the association, sometimes to participate actively in the overall administration, by a strong sense of solidarity.
- Persons with aphasia with severe disabilities (including physical impairments) who view the association as a meeting place and as a setting for a new lifestyle.

Family Members

Families of persons with aphasia make up another sizeable segment of the population in associations. Like persons with aphasia, they also do not form a homogeneous group. They can be categorized into two major subgroups.

- Family members who are actively involved on a regular basis in the overall organization of the association, yet who also attend to seek comfort among persons with similar experiences.
- Families who benefit from the services offered by the association to all members, e.g. social and cultural group activities, and information sessions on specific topics.

Therapists

The third group that can be observed within associations consists of therapists. Their role within the organization is usually linked to the founding of the association. Therefore, they occupy, over a fairly prolonged period, various functions: group leader, manager of the association, and liaison officer with the public.

Volunteers

Volunteers generally constitute a fourth group of members; their role is similar to that of the therapists.

Persons with Aphasia and Families who are Absent from the Associations

Associations currently serve only a few hundred of the tens of thousands of persons with aphasia living in Francophone countries. This circumstance is no doubt partly due to the recent emergence of these groups and the subsequent unawareness on the part of many persons with aphasia, therapists, and physicians of the existence of such associations.

Yet there are numerous persons with aphasia who have no desire to become members, and are even less inclined to participate in the association's activities. Apart from reasons of individual preference, there are several factors that may account for this lack of participation. An in-depth examination of these can lead to the formulation of improved arguments to persuade persons with aphasia to join associations in greater numbers.

Preservation of a Degree of Autonomy

Many persons with aphasia are elderly, and have already reached retirement age. They are often unmotivated, a result of the value which society attaches to work. They willingly and easily retreat into private activities. Moreover, their leisure activities are already organized and structured. If the symptoms of aphasia are not overly troublesome, participation in former activities will still be relatively feasible, and the persons will feel less of a need to seek out others or to look for new leisure activities.

Mr. V., for example, was employed at the time of his stroke. The nature of his job, however, was such that he used to spend afternoons in a social center where he engaged in group activities. Although the effects of his hemiplegia preclude participation in certain games requiring fine motor skills, his marked aphasia does not prevent him from participating in other activities that better suit his capacities. Thus all efforts to recruit him to the association have been fruitless.

Severity of the Disabilities

A certain proportion, unfortunately a significant one, of persons with aphasia experience severe lingering physical and linguistic impairments. It is quite understandable that these severely-disabled persons are hardly interested in joining an association, were it not for reasons of solidarity. They are confronted with a harsh reality: Dependence on others. Absence of loved ones and of resource persons and considerable difficulties finding accessible transport restrict these patients' mobility.

Physical Barriers

Sometimes hemiplegia alone limits the mobility of persons who would otherwise enjoy belonging to an association. Even the architecture of certain housing (e.g. lack of an elevator) virtually imprisons some people. They are cut off from any social interaction, aside from the isolation imposed by their language deficits. Another major problem is the lack of accessible transport, described above.

Distance

Some persons with aphasia live too far from the associations' meeting places. This is particularly true for those who live outside major cities. The travel involved, even if possible, is often too demanding to be undertaken on a regular basis.

The Need to Forget

Aphasia is not always a permanent disability. Those who are fortunate enough to experience a sufficient regression of their symptoms sometimes tend, acting on an all too natural reflex, to shun anything that reminds them of their traumatic experience.

The Fear of Being Judged by Society

Many persons with aphasia refuse this social contact because they are ashamed to be labelled a "disabled person."

Naturally, it is quite rare for a relative of a person with aphasia to participate in an association's activities on his own. The above mentioned barriers that deter the participation of persons with aphasia also affect the number of family members who become involved with associations.

OBJECTIVES AND ACTIVITIES

Each association engages in somewhat different activities owing to its history, geographical location, recruitment, and directors. These activities are also determined by the objectives behind the group's creation.

When an association is founded, the organizers must draw up legal documents. The wording of these differs according to the law in effect in each country. Yet each docment, whether it is an official charter, license, legal name, or any other document, generally describes the principal objectives of the group. By reading them, we discern that associations for persons with aphasia tend to share largely similar objectives. Here is a non-exhaustive list:

- to help the persons and their families escape their isolation and help one another;
- to help members learn to derive pleasure from life, once again, and to regain the desire to communicate;
- to promote social, professional, and familial reintegration;

- to provide information, and to solve legal and administrative problems;
- to raise public awareness of the difficulties faced by persons with aphasia;
- to gain recognition of aphasia as a disability;
- to defend the rights of persons with aphasia;
- to sensitize authorities and the general public to the needs of persons with aphasia;
- to keep abreast of, and to stimulate, scientific research on aphasia.

The very names of certain associations[9] tend to represent their actual programs:

- in France, the Lyon association *RELAIS* [rencontre, expression, langage, activités, information, soutien] (meeting, expression, language, activities, information, support);
- also in France, the Clermont-Ferrand association *OASIS — Organisation des aphasiques pour le soutien, l'information et la solidarité* (Organization providing support, information and solidarity for persons with aphasia).

Moreover, the titles of certain publications of associations[9] also evoke their group spirit. For example:

- *Se comprendre* [Understanding One Another] (Association for persons with aphasia — Brussels, Belgium);
- *L'Abri* [Shelter] (the Quebec Association for persons with aphasia —Montreal, Quebec, Canada);
- *La Jasette* [Chatterbox] (Association for people interested in aphasia — Quebec City, Quebec, Canada);
- *. . . et si cela vous arrivait . . .* [. . . and if this happened to you . . .] (National Federation of persons with aphasia in France — St-Germain des Fossés, France);
- *Sperantia* [Hope] (Association for persons with aphasia — San Miguel de Tucuman, Argentina).

These objectives, or rather statements of intention, can be categorized into five main themes which govern the association's activities. These themes are manifested in varying degrees, according to the association's operational priorities.

The Recreational Function

The recreational function of associations is undoubtedly the most universal one. It is the basis of most regular activities of associations in general.

The creation of independent and diverse leisure activities plays an important role in the development of the autonomy and social integration of persons with aphasia. Through role-playing and other games, and cultural activities, persons with aphasia can renew contact with themselves and with others. They can subsequently rediscover their abilities, mobility, sense of humor, and much more.

Solidarity

Solidarity is a key element in associations, for persons with aphasia as well as for their families. Most often, the appearance of this tragic event (the illness) in a family, and particularly in a couple, creates a severe and quite justifiable disequilibrium. Family members may have specific questions in mind: Administrative duties are often difficult to grasp. They also need to talk about their upheaval, their anguish, and their hopes. Neither physicians, nor social workers, psychologists, or even speech pathologists are entirely qualified to answer their questions. Yet those who have experienced living and coping with this trauma can be of significant assistance in satisfying family members' quest for answers. Families find each other during the persons' recreational activities, they share their experiences and support each other. This enables them to overcome, if not the suffering that can only be shared, at least the material difficulties that may arise. There, spouses can find a release for the communication that is lacking with their partners. They find an eager, attentive, and calm audience for their worries, their questions, and their daily difficulties. Members learn together, hope together, mourn the loss of language together, rejoice together, and discuss just about every issue dealing with the spouse and the person's daily existence.

Expressed differently, but for similar reasons, bonds of solidarity can also be observed within a group of persons with aphasia. For example, there is an emphasis on exchanging information and on offering encouragement. Members bring to meetings documents that they would like to understand better, forms to fill out, and mail to be answered. They phone each other regularly to keep in touch and to make sure that everyone is alright. They visit each other as well.

The Quasi-Therapeutic Role

The quasi-therapeutic role has been discussed above in the section dealing with the creation of associations. It consists in restoring the confidence of persons with aphasia by allowing them to speak among themselves and with other members, for example spouses of persons with aphasia, in an exclusive, comforting, and sheltered environment. This provides a preview of the reimmersion into society in general. Such objectives are particularly evident when an association chooses to be located in a medical or paramedical facility, a decision which may stem from *non-acceptance* of the termination of therapy. However, if we view the group's orientation in a more positive light, we can conclude that, overall, it represents a sincere desire to preserve the potential for communication acquired so laboriously during treatment — quite a legitimate aspiration.

The therapeutic role is evident in exercises to stimulate language, which are proposed during regular meetings with persons with aphasia, or printed in the association's newsletter. These exercises usually originate from a data bank diligently compiled by a counsellor or even by a person with aphasia working with therapists (speech pathologists or psychologists) who are known to the group.

Publicizing Aphasia

The necessary task of explaining aphasia in society has been outlined in Chapter 12. To combat indifference, rejection, and deprecation which constitute the most common reactions in society towards persons with aphasia, there is a need to clarify the syndrome and its consequences. It goes without saying that associations are particularly well-placed to disseminate this information. A variety of publicity media are used: newspaper articles, videos, conferences, radio programs, meetings with physicians and politicians, scientific information sessions, and national and international conventions.

The attainment of this goal — raising awareness on aphasia — proves to be particularly painstaking due to the dominant ideology that does not recognize aphasia as a disability. Furthermore, society is not interested in the problem. Must we wait until a celebrity acquires aphasia for the problem to finally interest the media and attract greater attention from the public?

The goal to better educate the public has included events such as the emergence of national federations in France and Belgium, the planned creation of an international federation of associations for persons with aphasia, the founding in the United States and Canada (and let us hope elsewhere in the near future) of an annual aphasia awareness week. These events all confirm the substantial and growing interest in this cause. Unfortunately there is still a long way to go before the general public becomes fully aware of the painful saga of the brutal onset of aphasia.

Defense of the Rights of Persons with Aphasia and their Families

This last theme is directed at federations of associations, since we are referring to national, rather than local, objectives. The goal here is to achieve recognition of aphasia as a deficit in itself, and not as a syndrome simply associated with hemiplegia. This is a logical progression from the consciousness raising described above. Beyond the legal and financial implications, there is a need for a humane appreciation of this severe disability.

The introduction of identity cards for persons with aphasia (Figure 16–1) clearly illustrates this well-founded battle with political and social authorities for the recognition of aphasia as a specific disability. The card indicates, in a succinct and personalized manner, that its carrier has communication disturbances impairing comprehension, expression, reading, and writing (the irrelevant disabilities are crossed out). It has no legal value. In France, for example, there is an official disability card. Yet the card contains no mention of the specific problem. The existence of a card designed exclusively for persons with aphasia can clarify for listeners the nature of the problem, thus avoiding situations where the person with aphasia is mistaken for an individual who is drunk, drugged, or even mentally deficient.

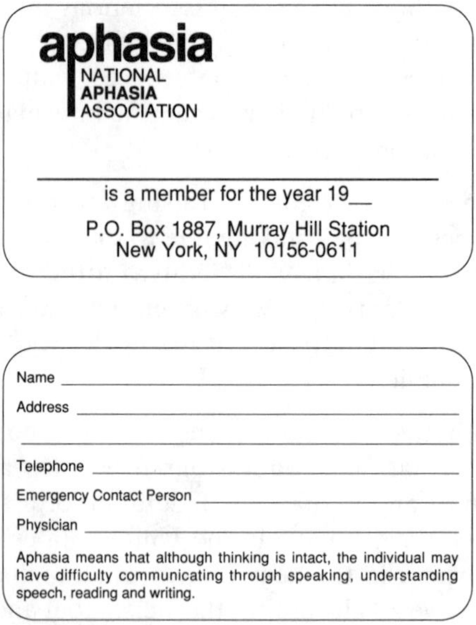

aphasia
NATIONAL
APHASIA
ASSOCIATION

____
is a member for the year 19__

P.O. Box 1887, Murray Hill Station
New York, NY 10156-0611

Name ________________

Address ________________

Telephone ________________

Emergency Contact Person ________________

Physician ________________

Aphasia means that although thinking is intact, the individual may have difficulty communicating through speaking, understanding speech, reading and writing.

Membership card of the National Aphasia Association

Figure 16–1

At the “First International Conference of Associations for Persons with Aphasia”[7], to which we referred at the beginning of the chapter, several national associations shared their views on the existence and value of such cards within their organization.

THE MANAGEMENT OF ASSOCIATIONS

Aside from the membership, objectives, and activities, associations for persons with aphasia and their families must also grapple with the issue of effective and official management. Usually operated as non-profit organizations, these associations require a team of directors who oversee the administration, coordination, and activities of the association.

Ensuring the survival of any association or similar group, in financial terms as well as through the coordination of services to the members, is an imposing challenge. This challenge is even greater when the members of the association all have language impairments. For example, how can they record the minutes at meetings? Who will draw up the bulletins and announcements? Who will be responsible for the accounting? Who will answer the phone? How can the group communicate with the public in order to promote awareness of aphasia? All these examples, and many others, amount to a painful and perpetual struggle for many persons with aphasia.

In general, associations tend to fall into one of three major categories of management systems.

Management by Persons with Aphasia

Some associations are managed entirely by persons with aphasia who regained language use to levels that closely correspond with their abilities before the illness. Many have recovered well; they represent, however, only 25 to 27% of the population with aphasia[5].

Occasionally, these individuals are fortunate enough to retain their jobs, with the understanding that they modify their work methods and their professional duties. They also attempt to adapt to the effects of aphasia lingering despite a so-called optimal recovery.

Within the organization, they represent the managerial core, and they fully administer the association. At times, during specific transactions, they must solicit external help. Nonetheless, whatever the task at hand, they demonstrate an ever-present desire to preserve autonomy in their operations.

Note that this type of management structure is, unfortunately, not predominant in the majority of associations currently in existence. In fact, among the persons with aphasia who are members of an association or support group it is rare to observe those who are capable of taking on such extensive responsibilities. Experience has shown that the individuals who are best suited for these roles tend to avoid the association for fear of being categorized as *disabled.*

Shared Responsibilities

This is a more commonly seen type of management in associations. The administrative duties are fairly and effectively shared between persons with aphasia, their families, therapists, and volunteers. The board of directors typically includes representatives from the first two categories of members. Therapists and volunteers may also join the organizers of the association as administrators or as resource people.

The board of directors of these organizations is usually composed in the following ways:

- the majority of the directors are persons with aphasia;
- the majority of the directors are family members of the persons with aphasia.

The effectiveness of the format chosen hinges on respect, confidence, and loyalty. As we have already mentioned, this type of management is characteristic of a greater number of associations. We also must add that each association has its own particular overall organization. Depending on the association:

- a person with aphasia and a family member may be responsible for accounting;
- a person with aphasia and a volunteer may coordinate the leisure activities;
- an extended board of directors may exist, in which therapists and volunteers play an active role;
- an extended board of directors may be present, characterized by the regular attendance of all the people responsible for files, committees, and activities.

The Role of Therapists

The third type of management is similar to the preceding one. Yet, in this system, therapists tend to play dominant roles in the creation of the association and the implementation of the administrative structure (coordination, finance, and overall orientation).

The prominence of the therapists' role gradually diminishes, to give way to a management system outlined in the section on "shared responsibilities." In contrast, although this type of management model may be found in several associations, each group will have specific agendas regarding the duration of the transitional period between the two types of management.

In general, we can describe most of the known associations with reference to the diagram below (Figure 16–2):

THE FUTURE OF ASSOCIATIONS

Two concrete issues determine the general evolution of associations for persons with aphasia. First and foremost, at the local level, each group is shaped by specific characteristics such as its various activities; these will be influential factors in its development. Secondly, organizations with national or even international scope can undertake collective activities that reach a wider audience. Consciousness-raising campaigns aimed at government authorities and the public, national or international conventions, promotional campaigns, and the defence of the rights of persons with aphasia are all activities which demand a certain official collaboration so that the energies furnished by each association will bring about results. At any rate, progress within associations, in spite of this dual reality, is often coupled with certain challenges which must be taken into consideration.

Financial Autonomy

First and foremost lies the issue of financial autonomy which allows the association to fulfill its commitment to all its members to the greatest extent. In any group, the available funds usually originate from several sources: membership cards, individual or corporate donations,

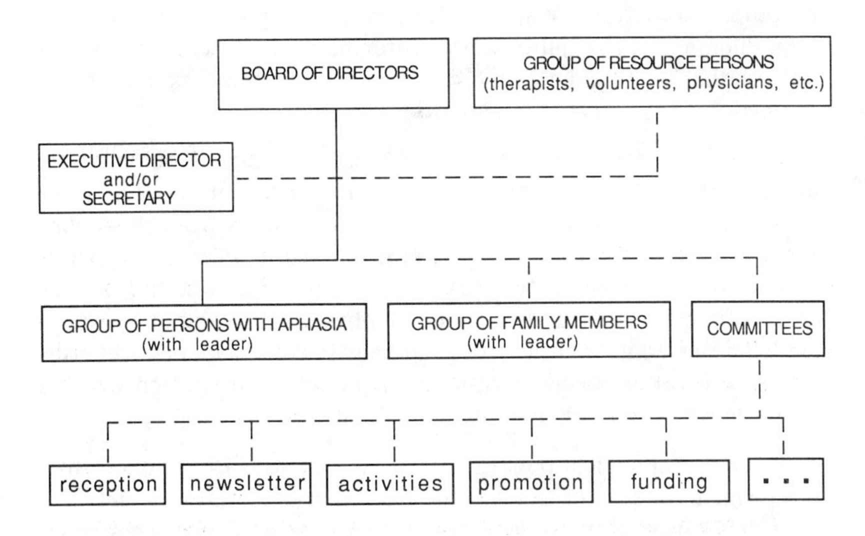

Association Tree

Figure 16–2

government subsidies, or from the movement's own fund-raising efforts. Generally an association's financing continues to be largely based on the first two sources on our list. The political orientations of the governments presently in power tend to encourage the privatization of social groups, since government subsidies are increasingly difficult to obtain. Apart from the reams of paperwork required, to operate, successfully, an association, organizers must resort to an array of fund-raising strategies. To cover all their needs, they appeal to several government organizations. Each financial *backer* imposes strict selection criteria, and requires the applicant to specify clearly the way in which the subsidy would be spent. When an association manages to find the necessary human resources to complete these administrative procedures, the financial support obtained often proves to be altogether insufficient.

As a result, the paucity of resources and the scarcity of subsidies stunt the growth of the majority of associations, despite the pressing need by members for support and the spread of information. The groups are forced, despite themselves, to assign priorities to their regular activities, retaining as their chief and often sole objective the provision of direct services to their members, a goal which can often be achieved at a minimal cost.

Human Interaction

The second challenge revolves around human interaction within the group. Coexistence between persons with aphasia, their families, and others who are interested in aphasia raises, quite understandably, many dilemmas. Associations, no matter how small, seek operational methods that will maximize the capacities of all members, taking into account, of course, individual limitations.

Each group determines the type of members who will belong to the association. However, regardless of the decisions made by the founders, the effectiveness of the association stems from its general philosophy, and from each of its members. Each member is entitled to the same benefits when he or she joins an association, whether the person is a therapist, researcher, student, physician, or someone who is simply interested in aphasia. Everyone may become a member in order to receive or offer specific assistance. In addition, it is often the case that those who offer help later become the recipients.

From a sociological perspective, all associations form "micro-societies" which are subject to the same rules that exist within society as a whole. It is reasonable to believe, however, that the challenge of communication occupies a particular position within an association for persons with aphasia. After all, is human interaction not based on *communication*?

Management of the Association

The administration, the programming, the coordination, in a word, the management of associations, constitutes the third challenge. Every association aspires to achieve a logical and effective coordination of the human and the financial resources at its disposal while it attempts to fulfils its primary objectives. Another major goal is to find a management system that will, above all, meet the members' needs most adequately, while simultaneously protecting the rights and interests of persons with aphasia and their families.

Contingent upon the association's other two challenges, effective and comprehensive management of each group must take into account the available financial means and human resources, that is, the people that are willing to participate in the management of the association. As in any business, adequate management is considered an indispensable asset which promotes the development and survival of the organization. Two main questions raised by the third challenge are *who* should be responsible for management, and *how* should this responsibility be assumed.

Most associations resolve these issues by establishing administrative structures consisting of a president and a board of directors. As witnessed in the histories of associations on record, the establishment of these structures is based, in the early stages, on the efforts of volunteers. The fragility of this procedure later obligates associations to seek more stable solutions; it is then that "executive" positions emerge, along with the notion of "permanence" within the group. The desire to offer a given remuneration to the individuals who fill these positions stem from the general management objectives. It clealy reflects the wish to guarantee long-term continuity within the association. Whether this mission be entrusted to a person with aphasia, an individual indirectly affected by aphasia, or simply a person who is aware of the problem, the goal of most associations is to attain maximal efficiency in their operations.

Apart from concerns about efficiency, these associations also value the presence of persons with aphasia (often a majority) in the board of directors and as case managers. Some associations develop management systems that are particularly interesting. Work teams are systematically composed of a person with aphasia and an able-bodied person. This approach, which can be aptly termed "pedagogical," allows for a certain "autonomization" of persons with aphasia who wish to participate actively in the management of the association. It is often the case that persons with aphasia, who are otherwise extremely active, are unable to accomplish certain tasks relating to management. Lack of self-confidence is often a hindrance to their involvement. The proposed work partnerships are proof of society's desire to evolve with regard to the acceptance and social integration of persons with aphasia.

Information

Lastly, in addition to the first three challenges, there is that of information. This affects members of associations, people affected directly and indirectly by aphasia, the general public, and various local, national, and international government bodies. Individually and collectively, associations must actively work to promote and defend the rights and interests of persons with aphasia and their families, while keeping in mind the limits imposed by the financial and human resources available.

The dissemination of information has a dual goal: To improve understanding and to demystify the nature of aphasia, on the one hand, and the person with aphasia, on the other. To do so, associations must produce various forms of publicity, hold conferences, and ensure widespread representation. It is up to each member to meet this challenge, whether they be a person with aphasia, a family member, therapist, physician, student, or merely a sympathizer. Each person plays an important role in the general and specific promotion of the association in the quest to achieve world recognition for this disability.

However, similarly to the requirements for effective management, the spread of information requires adequate and regular financing, as well as a significant amount of energy on the part of the human resources. For example, consider the expenses involved in the launching of the First International Aphasia Week which was initiated in June 1989 by the National Aphasia Association in the United States, and in which Quebec participated. We can only guess at the enormous sums required for the organization of the first international symposium, held in Belgium in 1989, that brought together persons with aphasia, their families, and representatives from the medical, paramedical, and technological fields[7]. According to the organizers, this event required considerable amounts of money, from the participants as well as from the association that organized this innovative event. Lastly, we would also like to mention that any consciousness-raising activities held in conjunction with the media represent a major challenge. To arouse interest in a topic like aphasia requires exceptional perseverance in any individual who dares to take on the task.

Each association meets these challenges according to its own capacities. In the Netherlands, for example, the launching of and support for associations for persons with aphasia form an integral part of the duties of therapists and the government. This decision by the authorities undoubtedly raises awareness of aphasia as a complex problem and boosts the quality of life in general and of services offered to persons with aphasia and their families. Note that, from a statistical standpoint, this government involvement directly contributes to the tabulation of precise data on the number of persons with aphasia.

CONCLUSION

Initiated ten years ago, associations for persons with aphasia are striving to carve out a place for themselves within society. The relevance of a social movement of this variety is now incontestable for every individual who wishes to promote universal medical and paramedical care. With regard to health care, for the past few years, legislative policies have been encouraging the creation of social movements in which persons with a medical problem can benefit from support groups of some kind.

Made up entirely of persons with aphasia and their families, these associations often owe their existence to the persistent efforts of therapists who believe in the necessity of rehabilitation within a more pragmatic context. Therapists are also present within the member population. They often occupy relatively key positions in the management sector of the association.

Local, regional, and national associations all aspire to increasing administrative stability, in order to ensure the necessary financial resources for the organization of their activities. This will subsequently enable them to fulfil their obligations towards their members and society.

Overall, associations are in the early stages of development. They still wage daily battles, and, to guarantee their survival, they actively combat problems in their overall management. Given the consequences of aphasia with which the persons must learn to cope, these challenges must not be underestimated.

Only recently have certain associations initiated attempts to promote, both locally and nationally, the rights and interests of persons with aphasia and their families. The recent formation of some European federations will certainly further this cause.

International movements are gradually emerging, and, during the first international convention of aphasia associations, the participants demonstrated their willingness to combine efforts in order to achieve recognition of aphasia as a specific disability.

To date, each association for persons with aphasia and their families is slowly progressing towards increased autonomy. Each group occupies an important, even primordial, place in the overall structure of a philanthropic movement that promotes full respect for persons with aphasia in their will to live again[(1)] and to reappropriate their own lives.

"When you break a leg, the long-term outcome is recovery; as long as there are no complications, it should take a few months. The fact that you can TALK to others is already HALF the healing process. When LANGUAGE is affected, it is much more difficult to SHARE the suffering with others.(. . .) The SUDDEN disappearance of language plunges us into a sea of despair, a depth of misery. The terror of an INEVITABLE void is INDESCRIBABLE . . . Can we one day escape from this yoke, this prison? We must trust immensely, and hope a great deal (. . .) With "Se Comprendre" (the Belgian association). I meet persons with aphasia who (. . .) take praiseworthy and bold INITIATIVES (. . .) These are persons with aphasia who show individual strength in the firmness of their decisions, and consistency in their performance, like a quantity of ENERGY."[8]

Words of HOPE for the Future: The Dreams of Persons with Aphasia

"That all persons can recognize their aphasia; it's not all kinds of strange things . . . it's aphasia. And later, with our friends at the association, it's still aphasia, but it's different, it's aphasia that can speak." (J.C.)

"I dream of a well-established association that will be highly respected. That will do spectacular things, major events. But . . . it should remain as humane as now, it should be people-oriented, people should come first." (F.P.)

"That those who see us in hospitals, physicians, recognize us, they should talk about and learn about aphasia." (N.B.)

"Maybe one day people will say . . . Perhaps the person has aphasia!" (L.M.)

"To have our own convention, one to which all the friends and family of persons with aphasia will be invited: Therapists, physicians, social workers, researchers, students . . . all together, because right now it's divided. We must think about helping each other, listening, and solving problems together. Oh yes! politicians too. You get it?" (R.D.)

"At first, a child, broken there (tilting his head to the left). But later, growing, growing, growing again, always. You have to. That's all." (G.G.)

REFERENCES

1. *Pour une meilleure qualité de vie dans son milieu.* Proceedings of the <<3e congrès canadien en réadaptation>>, Les éditions Papyrus, Québec, 1987.
2. Lecours, A.R., F. Lhermitte & Coll.: *L'aphasie,* Flammarion, Paris, 1979.
3. Cot, F. & Y. Joanette: *La rééducation en France vers 1900.* Document submitted for publication, 1990.
4. Ducarne de Ribaucourt, B.: *Rééducation sémiologique de l'aphasie,* Paris, Masson, 1986.

5. Ducarne de Ribaucourt, B.: Le Devenir des aphasiques. *Rev Neurol* (Paris), **136** (10): 617–628, 1980.
6. Ducarne de Ribaucourt, B. & F. Lhermitte: Problème psycho-logiques, sociaux et professionnels des aphasiques. L'Aphasique dans la société. *Evolution médicale,* **2:** 547–560, 1967.
7. *Premier Congrès International des Associations de Personnes Aphasiques et leurs Proches.* Proceedings of the conference, in preparation (held in Belgium, in 1989).
8. Association québécoise des personnes aphasiques & Coll.: *Paroles d'aphasiques.* Book in preparation.
9. Bassem, R. & M. Hubert: *Bottin international des associations pour personnes aphasiques.* Document in preparation.
10. Durieu, C.: *La rééducation des aphasiques*, Dessart, Brussels, 1969.
11. Seron, X.: *Aphasie et neuropsychologie,* Mardaga, Brussels,1979.